AF263985

Erotic Orient

Exoticism, fantasy, and sensual visions of the East

Hans-Jürgen Döpp

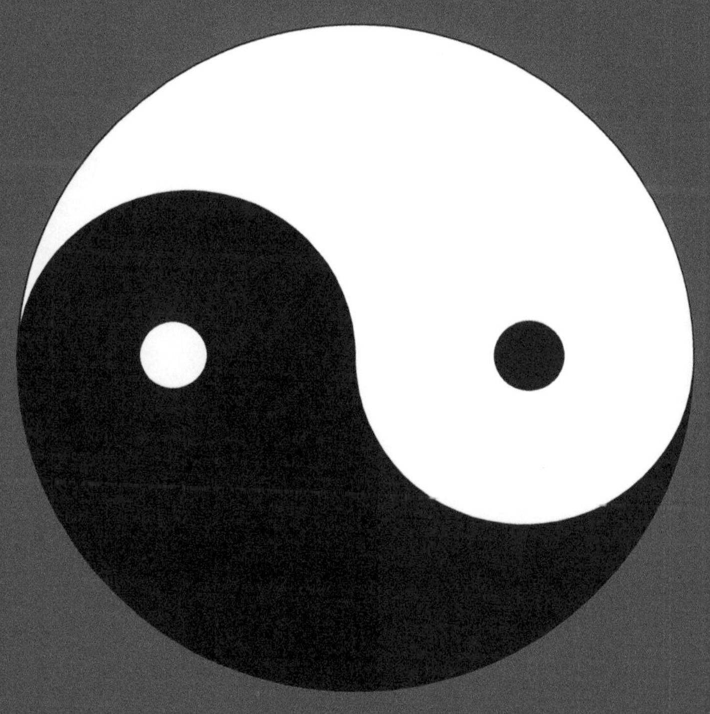

CHINESE EROTICISM

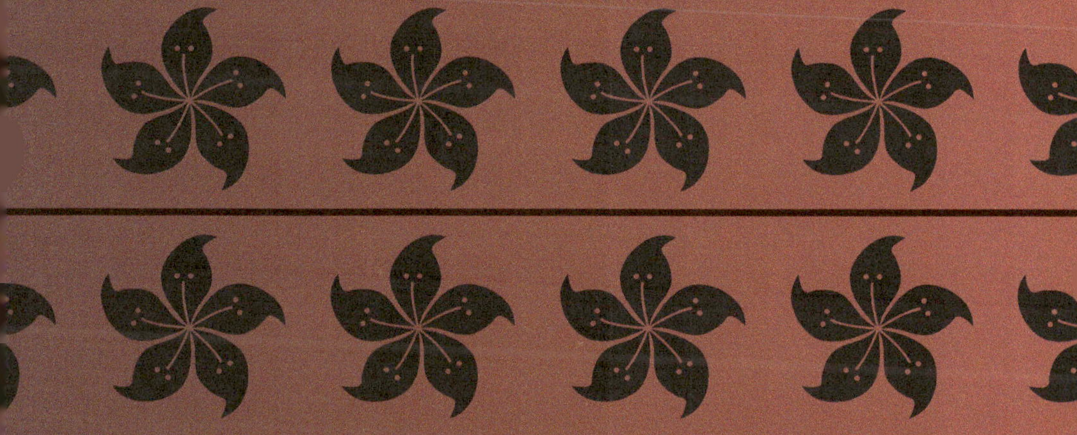

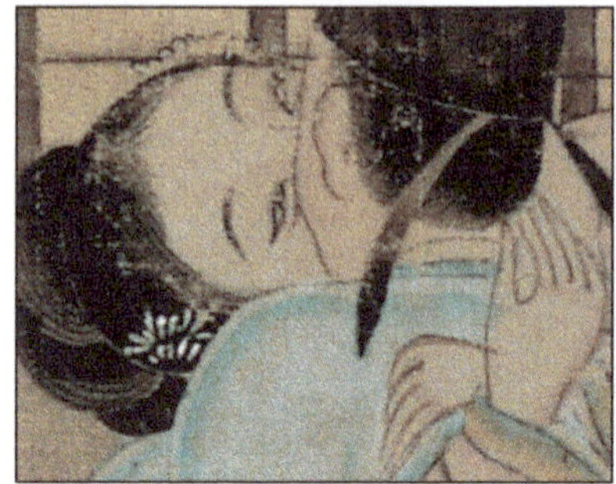

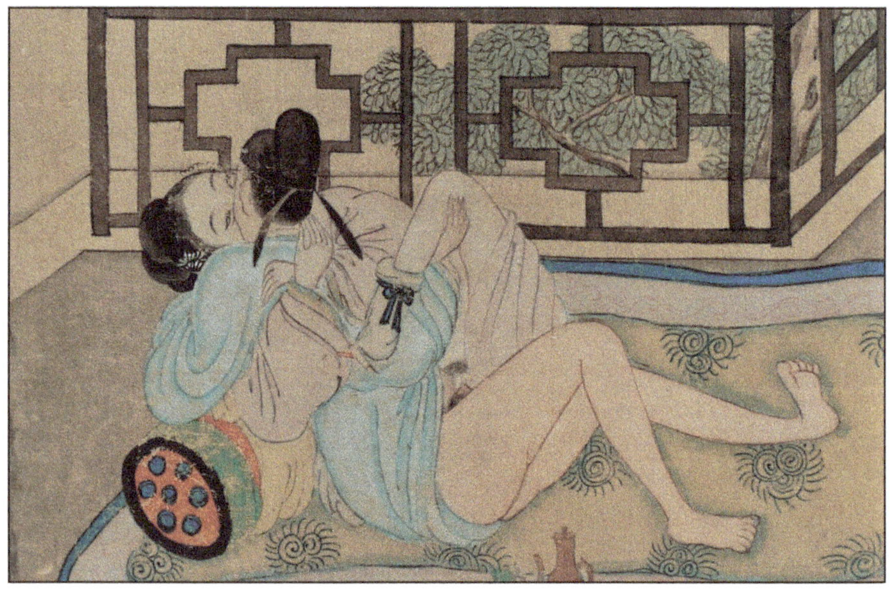

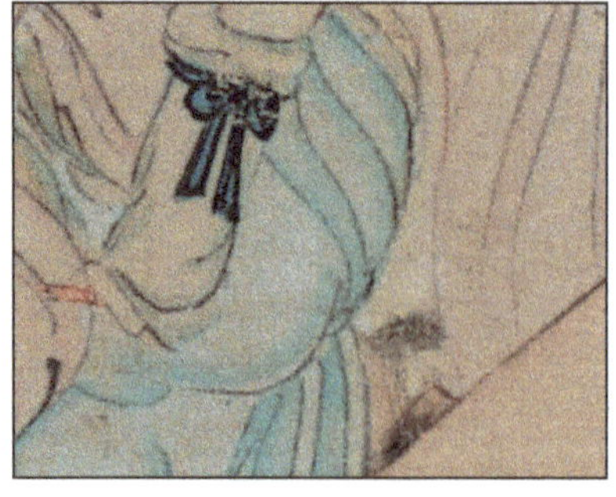

Bound happiness

Chinese eroticism

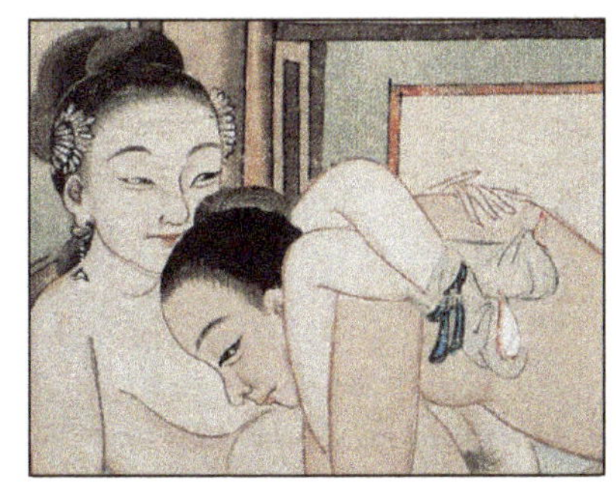

The aim of Taoist art and culture was to reach a state of harmony that would lead Man, confronted by a chaotic universe, towards a new serenity. In this spiritual context, love represented for the Chinese a force which was supposed to unite sky and earth in balance and maintain the reproductive cycle of nature. Eroticism thus became an art of living and formed an integral part of religion (to the extent that such western notions can be applied to philosophical thoughts of this kind).

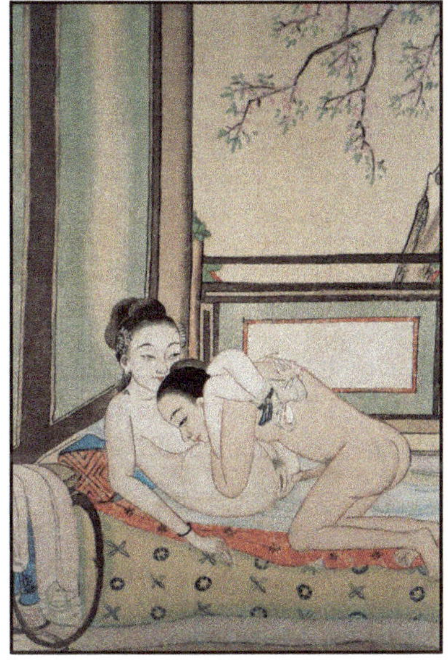

Taoist religion assumes that pleasure and love are pure. 'In order to gain some understanding of Chinese eroticism,' writes Etiemble, a great connoisseur of Chinese art, 'We need to distance ourselves from the notion of sin and the duality between the corrupt body and the holy spirit.' This ideology lies at the very base of Christianity. Erotic Chinese art reflects the extent to which we are 'morally corrupt' and 'full of prejudices.'

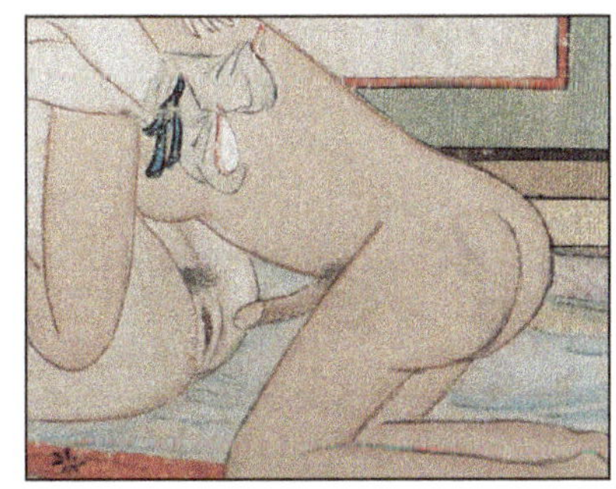

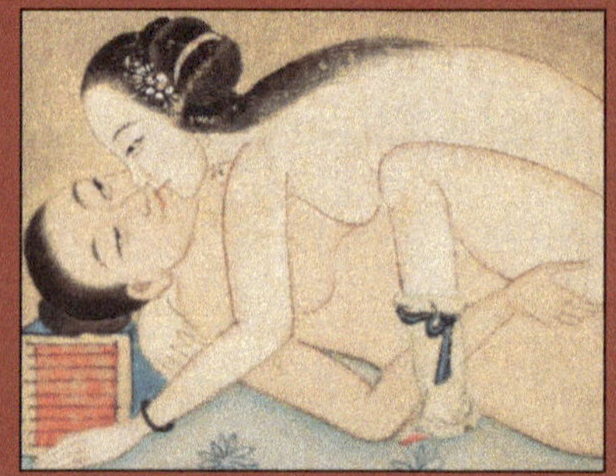

6

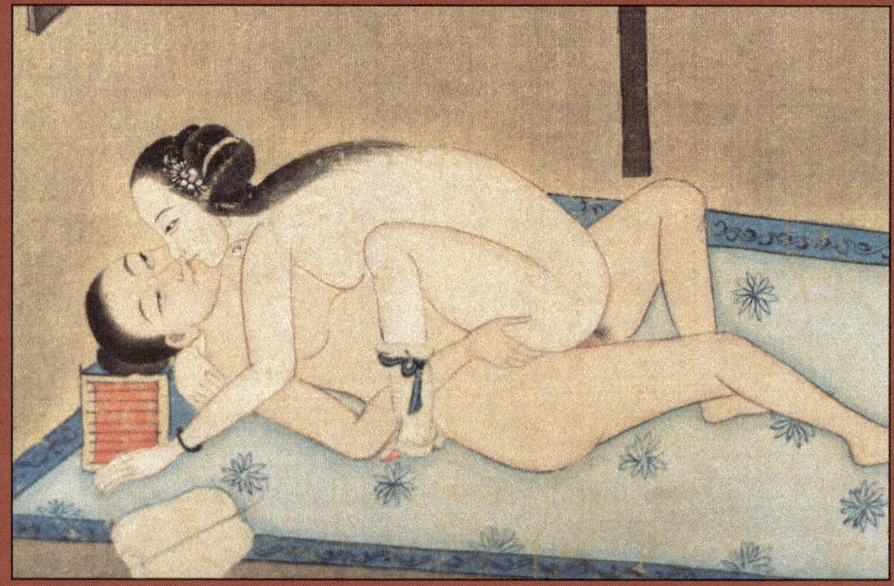

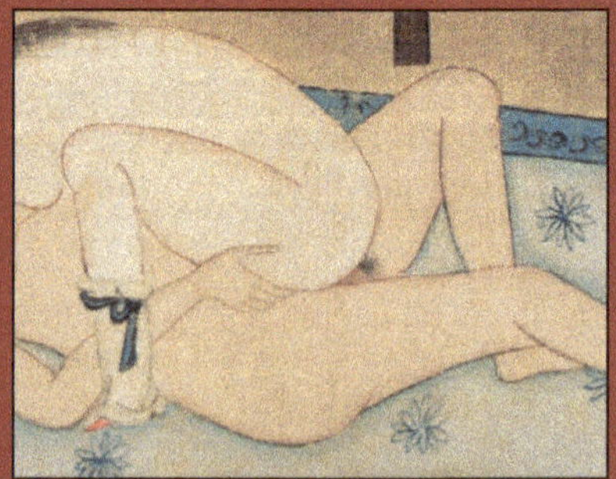

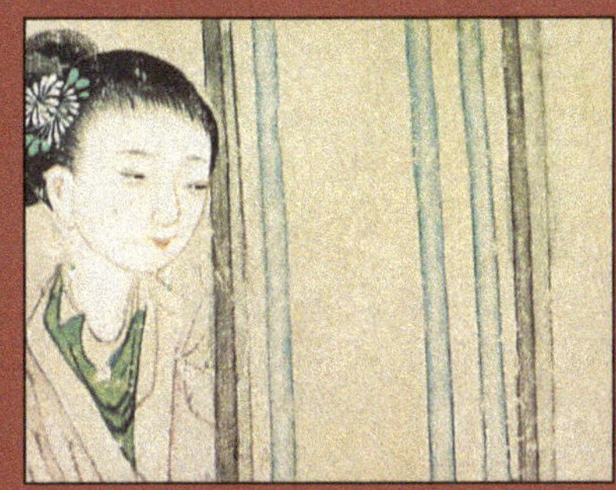

The Yin-Yang pairing introduces us directly into the world of Chinese eroticism: 'The path of Yin and Yang' signifies nothing less than the sexual act itself. One of the best-known sayings of ancient Chinese philosophy, 'Yi yin yi yang cheh we tao' ('On the one side yin, on the other yang, this is the essence of Tao') indicates the fact that sex between a man and a woman expresses the same harmony as the changes between day and night, or summer and winter. Sex symbolizes the order of the world, the moral order, while our culture stigmatizes it as evil.

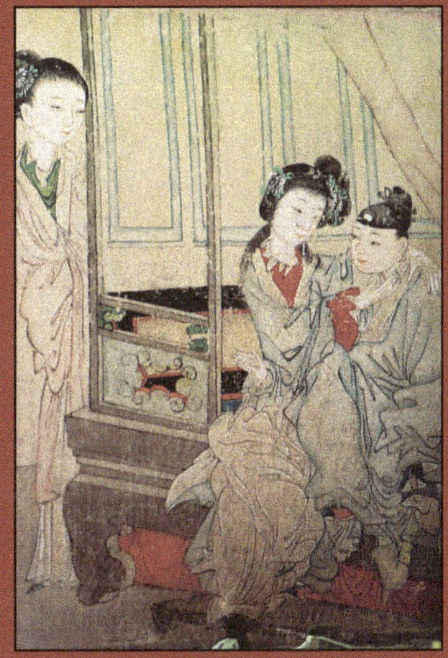

In this sense, master Tung-huan wrote in his Art of Love: 'Man is the most sublime creature under the skies. Nothing which he enjoys can be compared to the act of sexual union. Formulated according to the harmony between the sky and the earth, it rules Yin and dominates Yang. Those who understand the sense of these words can preserve their essence and prolong their life. Those who do not grasp their true significance are heading towards their doom.' The split in the Universe between Yin and Yang is all the more important because these two inseparable principles mutually influence each other.

7

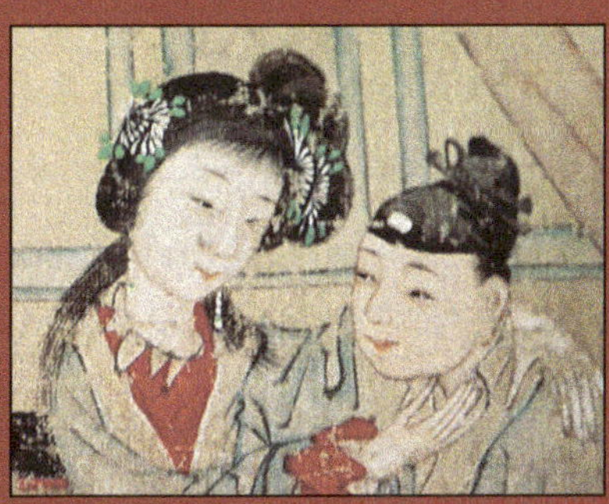

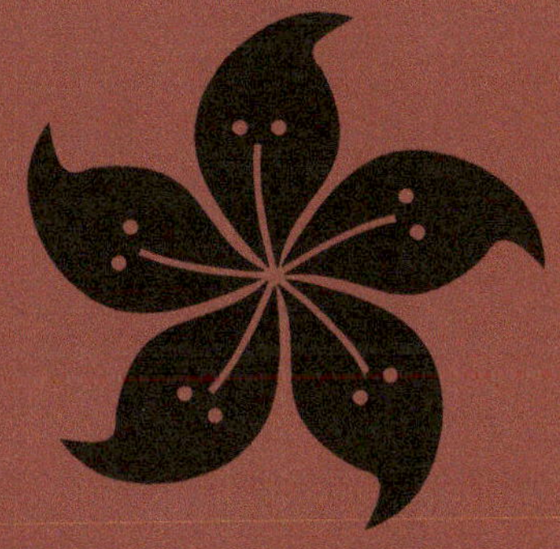

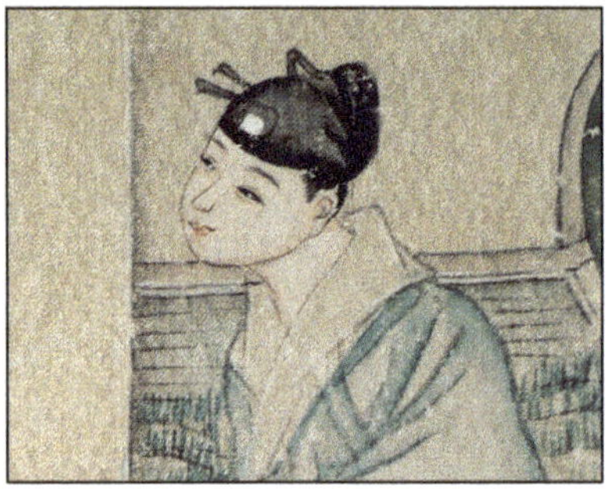

We know of a great many Chinese manuals whose purpose was to provide an education in the art of love-making for young couples; this education would cover desire, morality, and religion. In these texts, the sexual act is always referred to metaphorically, with terms such as 'the war of flowers,' 'lighting the great candle' or ' games of cloud and rain.' They are also full of images referring to various sexual positions:

- unfurling silk

- the curled-up dragon

- the union of kingfishers

- fluttering butterflies

- bamboo stalks at the altar

- the pair of dancing phoenixes

- the galloping tournament horse

- the leap of the white tiger

- cat and mouse in the same hole

8

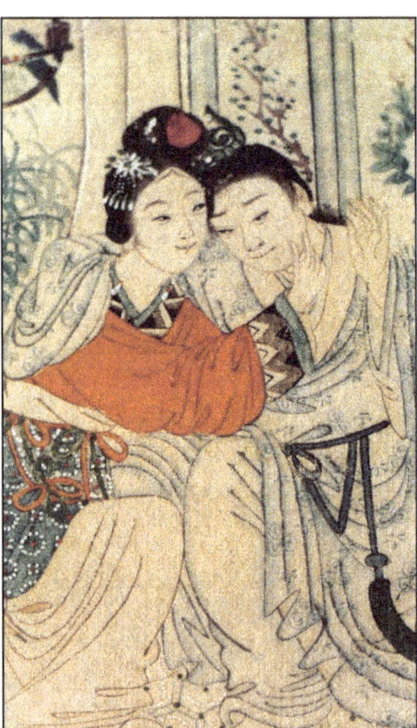

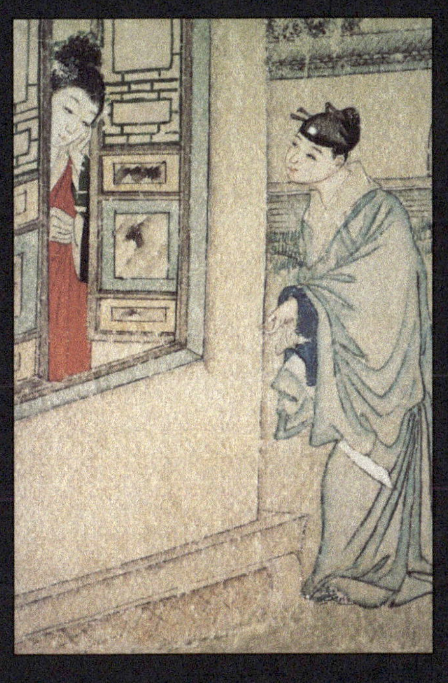

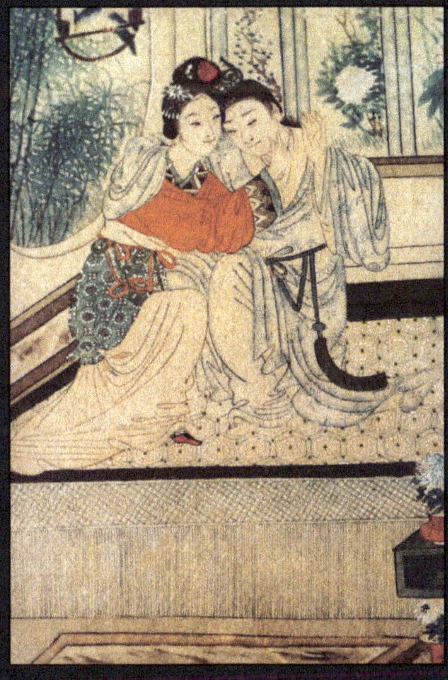

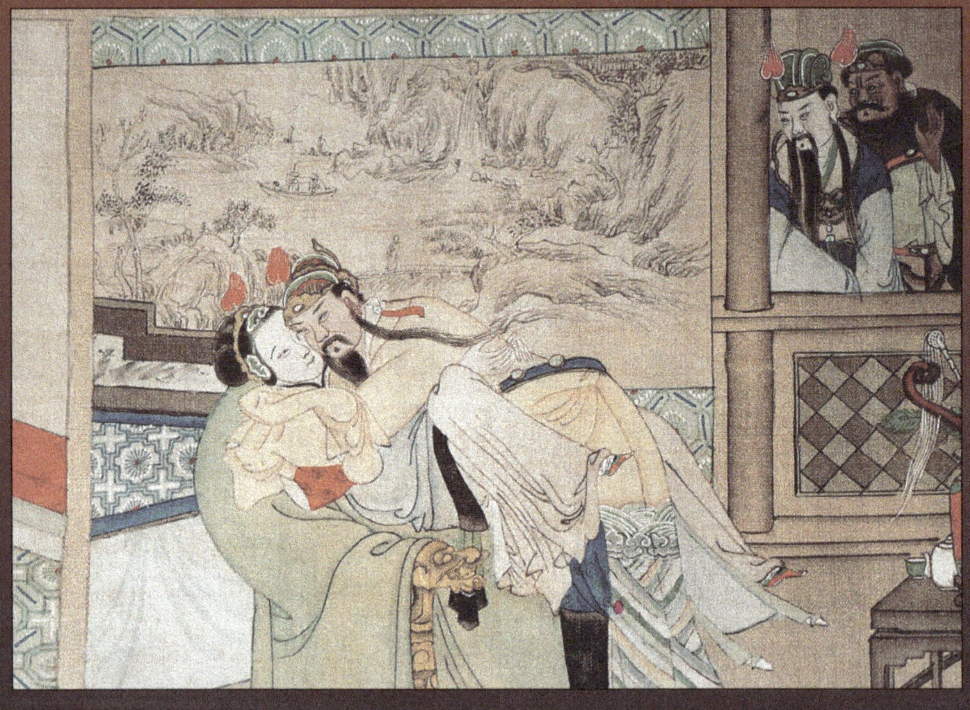

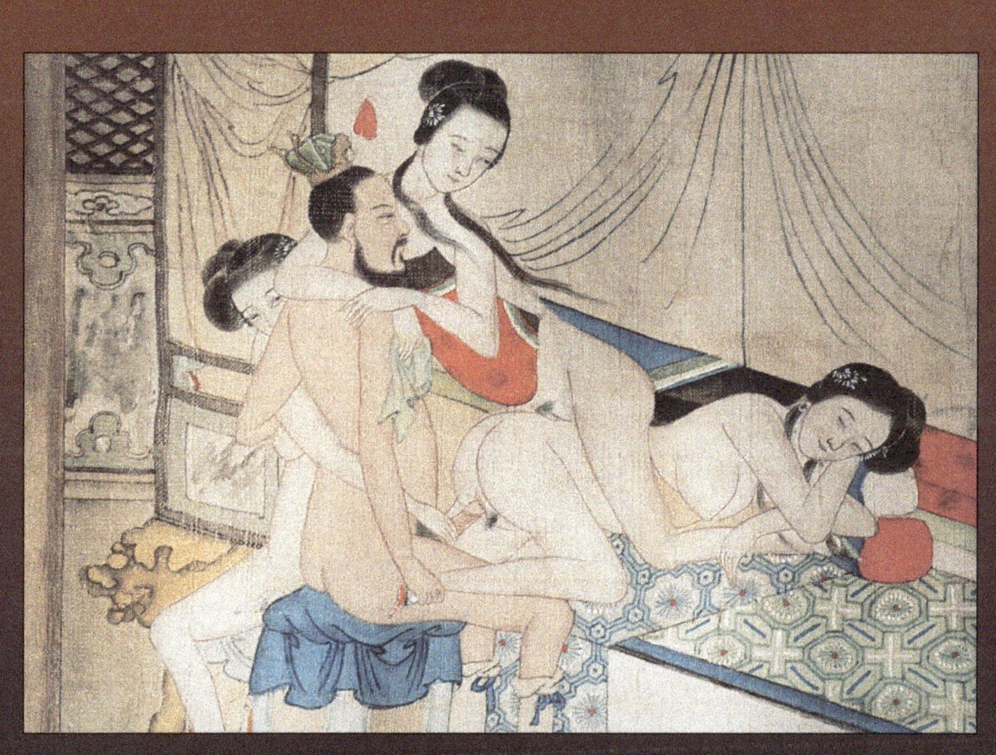

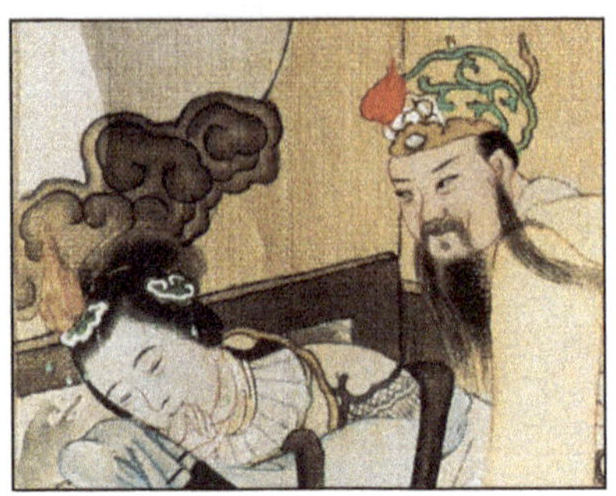

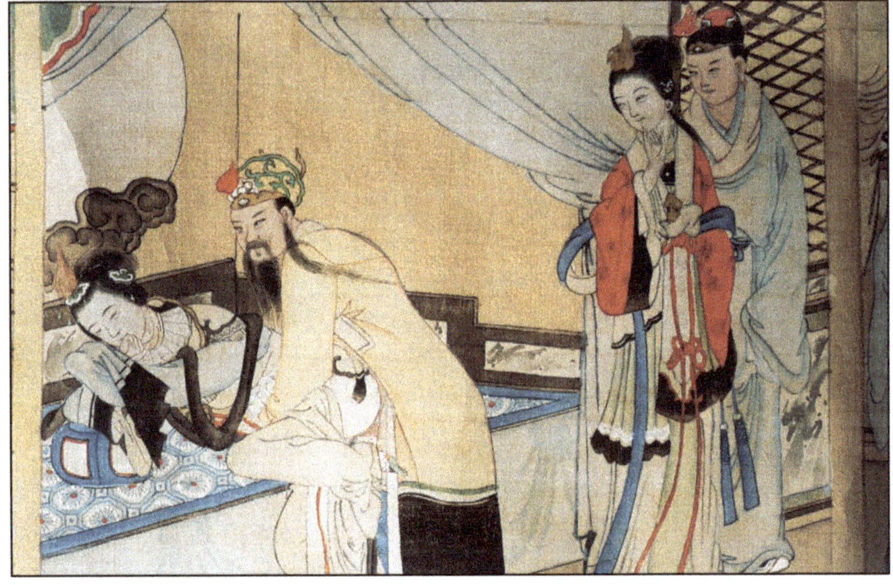

In Chinese aesthetics, nothing is ever named directly and without beating about the bush. Instead, things are referred to obliquely, and any transgression of this tradition is considered vulgar. Even the European notion of 'eroticism' would be too direct. They would prefer to substitute the term 'the idea of spring.'

Physical love is praised without pretence but also without vulgarity in the verses of a popular Chinese song:

'The window open in the light of an autumn moon,
The candle snuffed out, the silk tunic undone,
Her body swims in the scent of the tuberoses.'

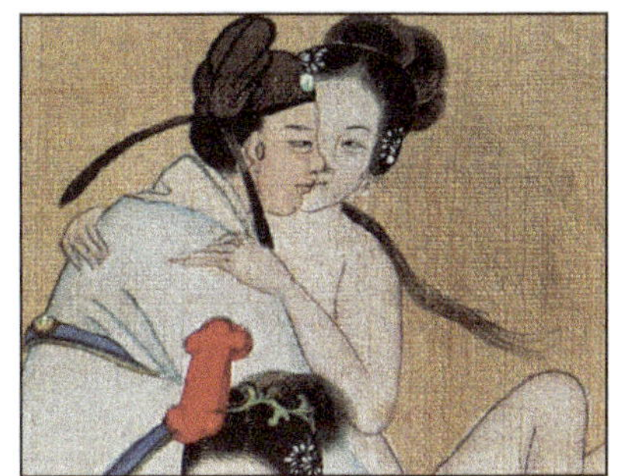

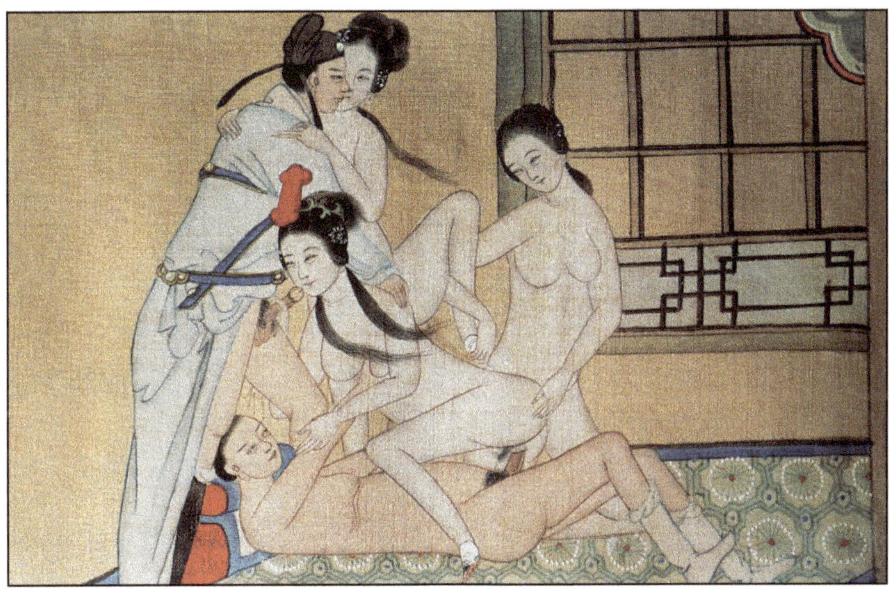

In the erotic images of paintings on silk or porcelain, wood engravings or illustrations, sexuality is never shown in its crude state or in a pornographic manner, but always in a context of beauty and harmony. Symbolic, meaningful details enrich these illustrations, evoking the tenderness which occupies a favoured place in Chinese iconography. Nevertheless, these details are difficult for Europeans to decipher: the cold and impassive faces of the lovers are a long way from our idea of a blaze of passion.

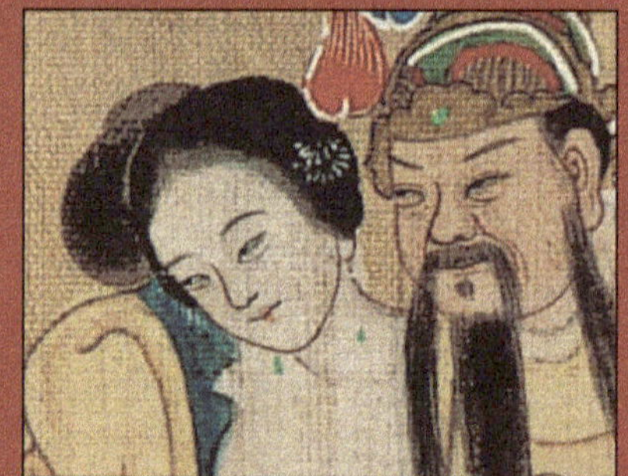

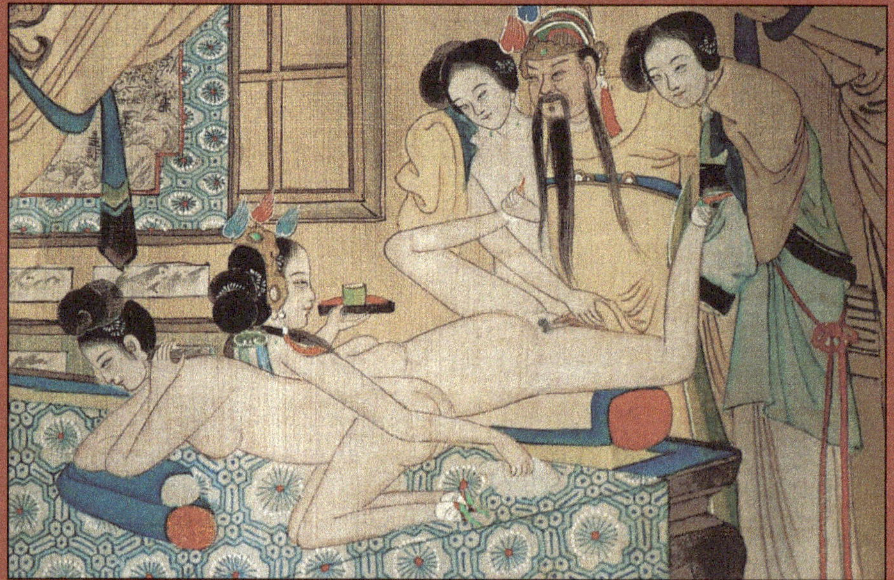

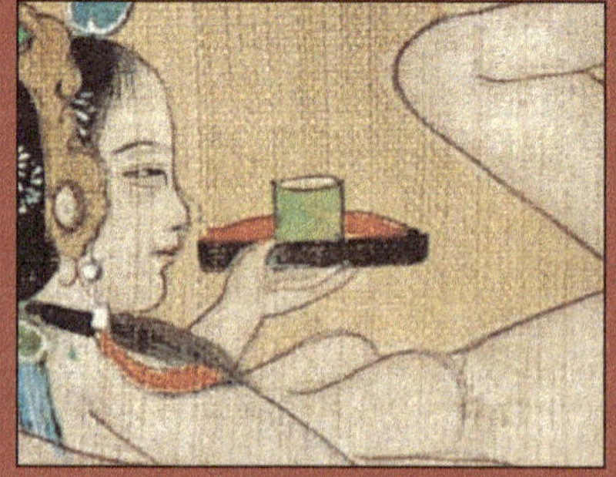

Thus it is that one of the most fertile and ancient cultures in the world invites us, through its religious practices, to make love. Taoist manuals advocate the technique of holding back from ejaculation, a truly prodigious invention which allows the man to satisfy the woman. By doing this, a subtle alchemy is achieved: the man receives Yin from the woman, who obtains from him the pure essence of Yang. For this reason, coitus reservatus is considered in Taoism and in Tantrism to be the most subtle form of sexual union, because it allows the crossing of the divide between masculine and feminine energy. The creation of a new life is not the principal aim of the sexual act. It has more to do with an identification with cosmic forces than with the forces of life.

The 'theory of juices' holds that sperm passes through the spinal column directly to the brain. During the 17th and 18th century, European medicine laboured under the same misapprehension. How painful it must have been to be a young boy masturbating and believing that doing so would lead to a degeneration of the spinal cord and a drying-out of the brain!

Whilst ejaculation provides a mere instant of pleasure which is very swiftly lost and finishes in the relaxation of the entire body, a buzzing in the ears, tiredness of the eyes and a dry throat, coitus reservatus or coitus interruptus provokes growth in vitality and an improvement in all the senses.

Among the best-known manuals are those of Sou Nu King and Sou Nu Fang, which among other things recount how the legendary Yellow Emperor, Huang-ti (2697-2599 B.C., according to traditional historical reckoning) used experienced women to teach him about the art of love-making. In The Treaties of the Bedroom there is a conversation between the Emperor and one of his mistresses, a simple young girl:

'The Yellow Emperor asks the simple young girl: My spirit is listless and lacking in substance; I live constantly in fear and my heart is full of sadness. What can I do to cure myself? The young girl replies quite simply: All human weaknesses come from an unhappy union of bodies during the sexual act. As water wins in the fight against fire, so woman gains in the fight against man. Those who are skilled in pleasure are like good cooks who know which five spices to add to a bowl of soup.

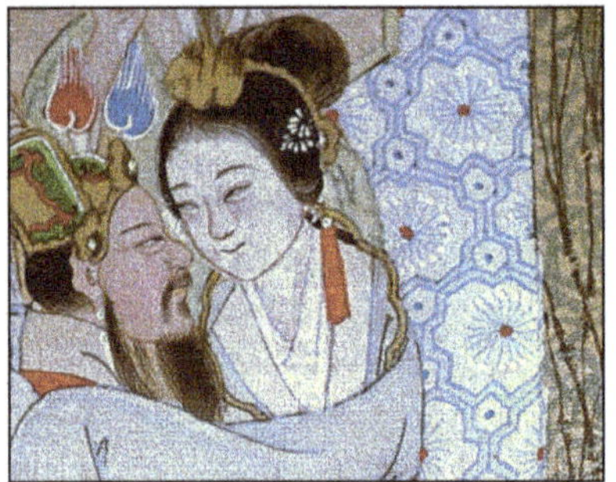

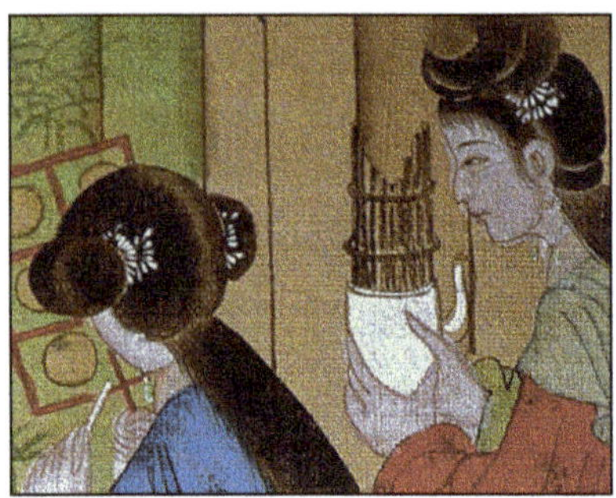

16

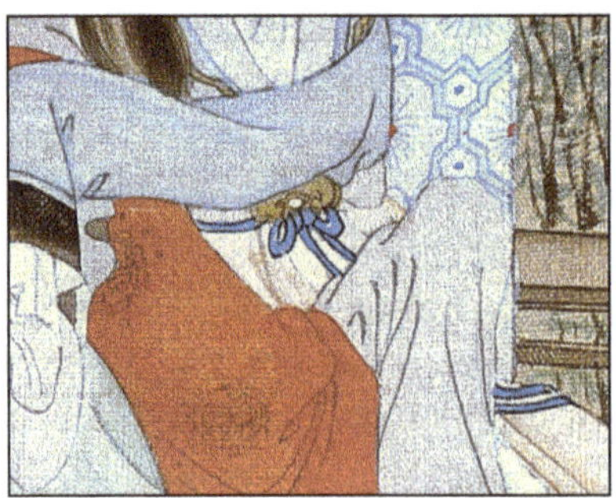

Those who understand the art of Yin and Yang can unite the five modes of pleasure; those who do not know this die before reaching the age of maturity and without having had the slightest pleasure from sex. Should one not forestall this danger?'

And in another lesson in the same work: Huang-ti asked: 'What does one gain from practising sex according to the path of Yin and Yang?'

'For man, sex makes his energies surge – for woman, it serves as protection against sickness. Those who do not know the right path think that the sexual act can be harmful to health. In truth, the sexual act has only one purpose: physical pleasure and joy, but also peace in the heart and strength of the will. The person feels neither sated nor hungry, he is neither hot nor cold; the body is satisfied and the spirit likewise. Energy ebbs and flows majestically, and no desire troubles this harmony. This is the result of a well-accomplished union. If one follows this rule, women will achieve full pleasure and men will always remain healthy.' Thus answered Sunu.

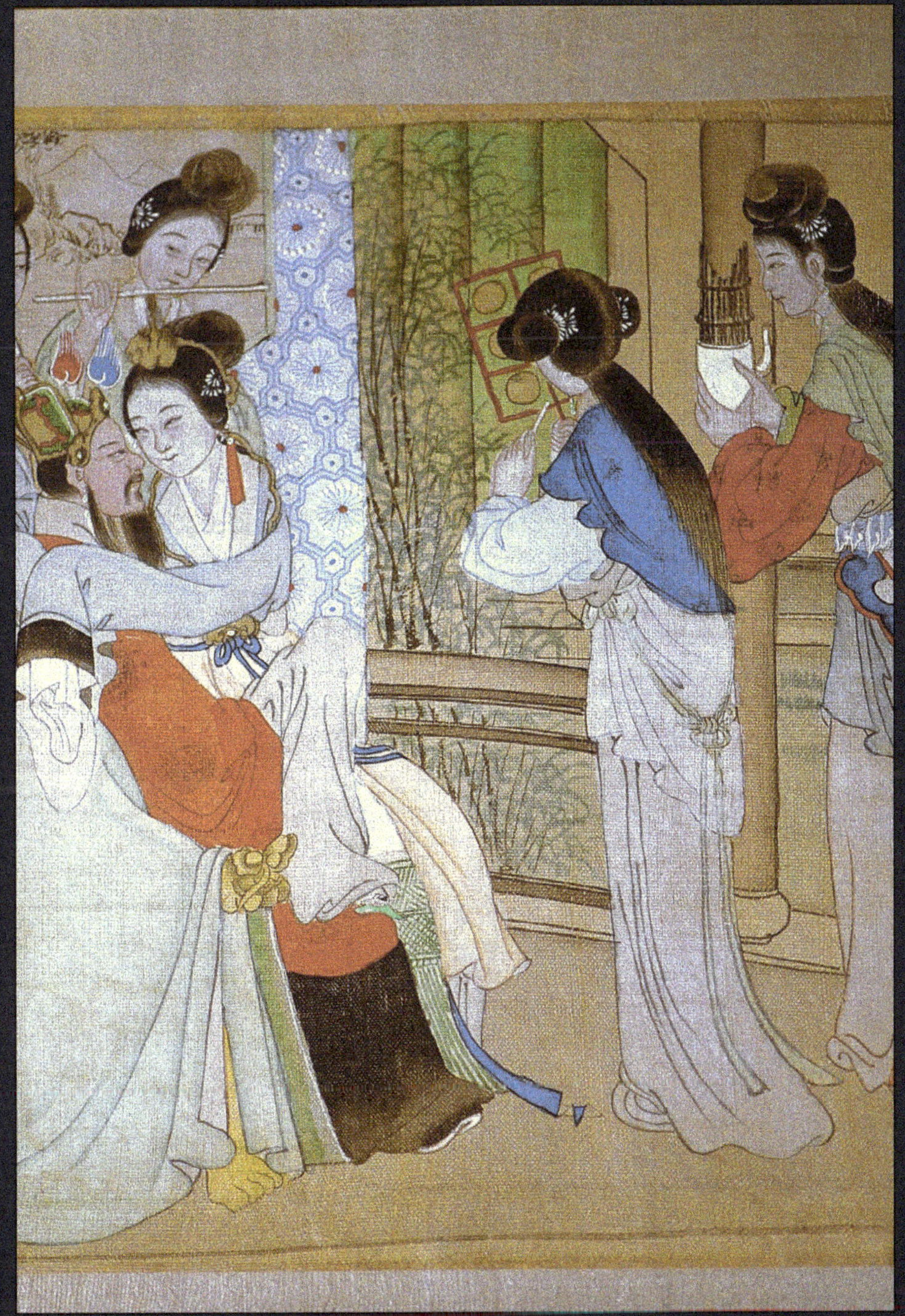

All of these manuals advocate
making love as often as possible
and even at an advanced age:
'Whatever his age, man would
not be happy living without a
woman. If he is without a
woman, his concentration suffers
because of it. If his
concentration suffers, the forces
of his mind grow weaker; if the
forces of his mind weaken, the
span of his life grows shorter…'

The bibliography of works of
the Han era, which is the era
directly pre-dating the birth of
Christ, includes eight books that
are entirely devoted to the art of
love-making. During that era the
following maxim was adopted:
'The art of having sexual
relations with a woman consists
of remaining master of oneself
and preventing ejaculation in
order to allow the sperm to
return to the brain.' From that
moment on, every educated
Chinese man felt obliged to be
familiar with the technique of
reinforcing masculine power
named 'drinking at the jade
fountain': the man had to remain
inside the woman while she had
her orgasm and only leave her
when it was over, without
releasing any sperm in the
process. The treatises teach that
it was even possible to make love
several times in one night with
different women if one followed
this technique. Taoist wisdom
emphasizes the positive aspects
of this for the man's health:

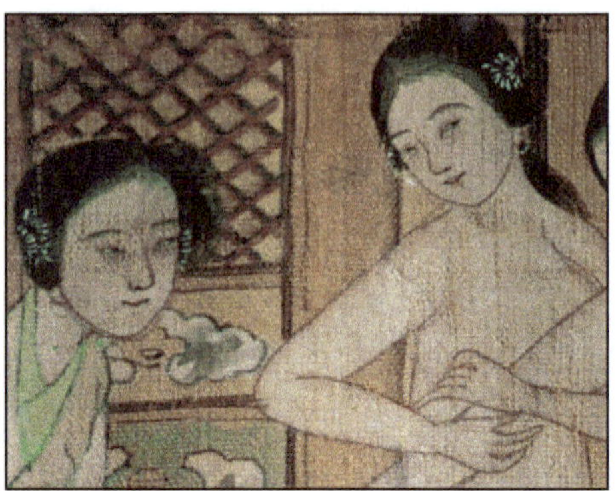

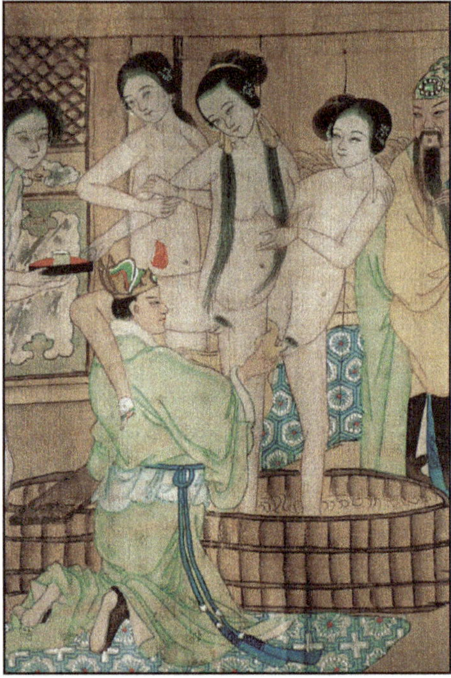

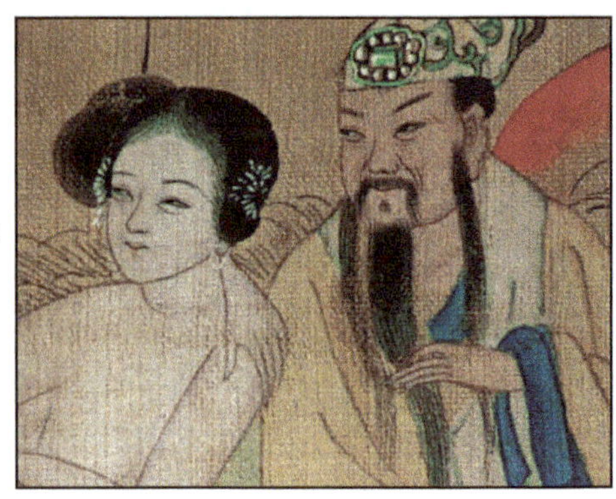

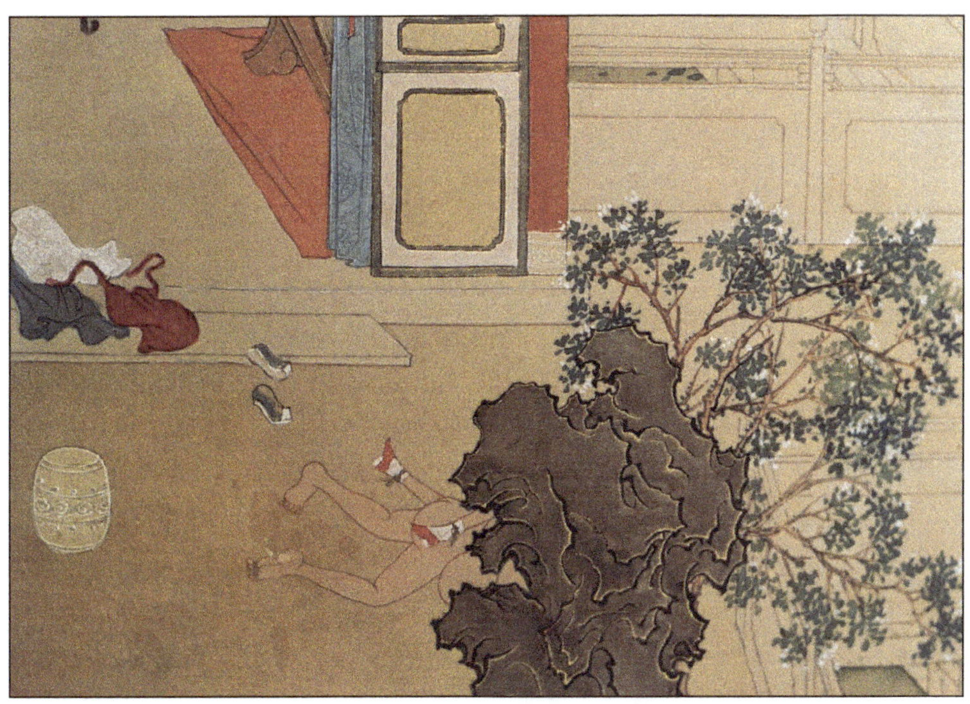

'Those who are capable of making love several times a day without spilling their sperm will be cured of all illnesses and will reach a ripe old age. If sexual relations are not limited to one woman, the success of this method will only be enhanced. The best option is to make love with ten women or more during the course of one night.'

Sex, medicine and religion are thus closely linked in Taoism because of the large number of energy channels that flow through the body. There is a link between the exterior world in which man lives and the individual interior of every human being. Sexuality is thus called upon to play a central role in everyone's life.

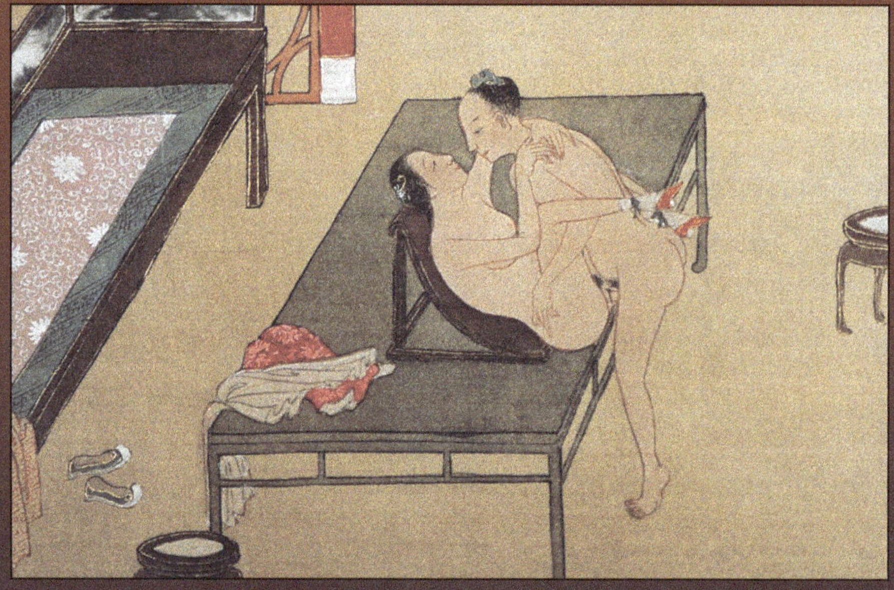

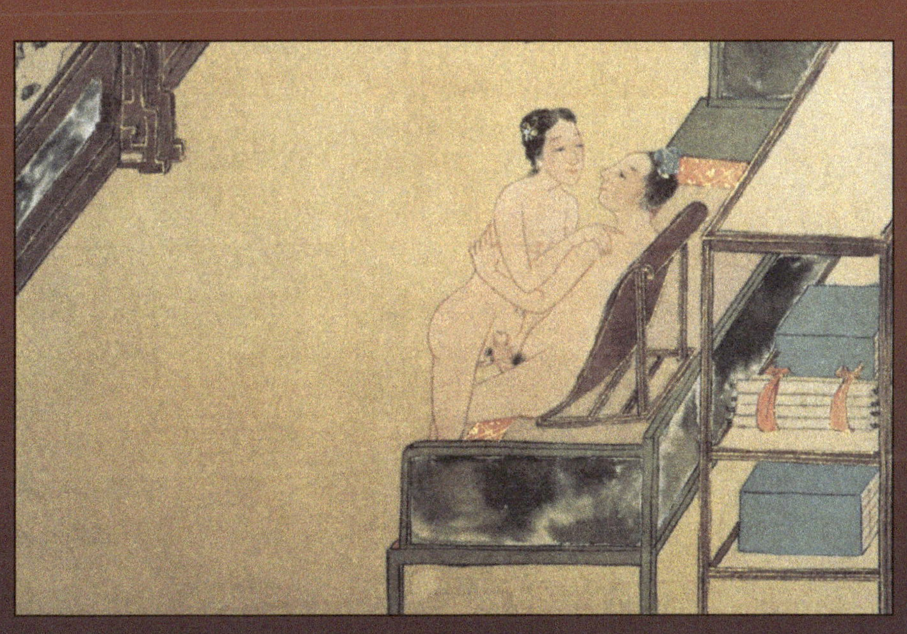

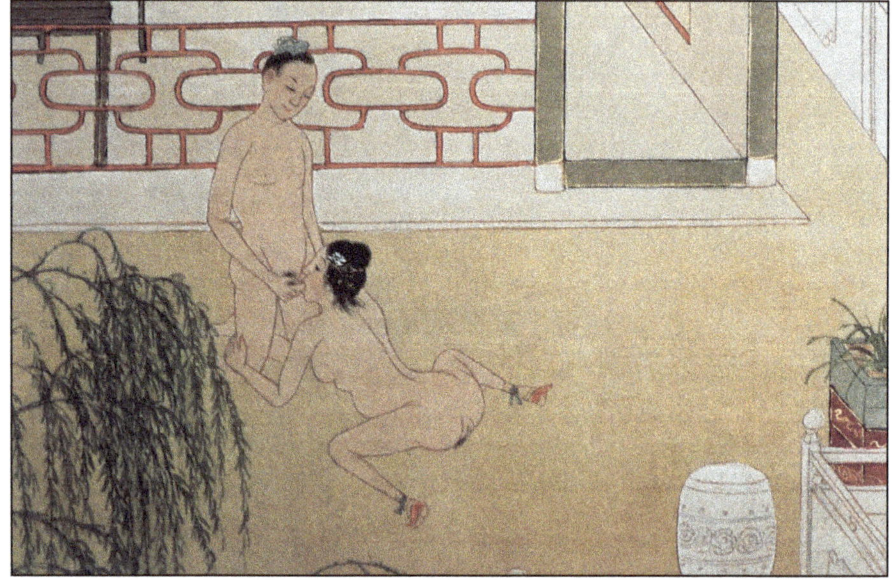

This explains why men thought of satisfying several women sexually as a duty. And the aim was to do it without exhausting all their energy. So, men were supposed to learn different erotic techniques for giving several women multiple orgasms without, however, experiencing their own.

Taoist education, from the simplest effort right up to the most elevated spiritual heights, was founded on the control of sexual energies.

Tantrism, influenced by Buddhism, was in its teachings and intentions largely similar to Taoism.

The greatest development in erotic art was principally concentrated in the rich commercial cities in the south of China, during the early part of the period that is considered the beginning of the modern era in Asia. From the 10th century onwards, cities as famous as Suzhou, Hanzhou or Quanzhou were among the most flourishing in the entire world. Businessmen frequented luxurious brothels, wine houses and other places of pleasure such as tea houses or the baths. They formed a sub-culture which today is largely documented by writings and novels from that period. The culture of courtesans was a part of this.

The golden age of Chinese erotic art dates from the end of the Ming period (1368-1644), which was characterized by relatively great liberty and the flourishing of all kinds of arts and science.

The prudery of Confucianism was the cause of the destruction of a great number of erotic paintings which illustrated the ancient Taoist manuals. Confucianism denied eroticism and advocated the separation of the sexes as well as the subordination of personal passions to the laws of family and the state.

Later on, Christianity played a negative role in favouring these iconoclastic practices. What had survived all of these eras was finally destroyed during the Maoist cultural revolution.

These philosophical detours can no doubt go some way to explain the delicacy of Chinese eroticism. Like a mantra, these pieces of information are repeated again and again in books about China. And yet Asian eroticism still remains very enigmatic to western understanding.

As Europeans, we cannot help but wonder how sexual ecstasy can be combined with a technique that is so precisely worked out and that is controlled by such a myriad of instructions and recommendations. Does it not lead to a loss of spontaneity in one's feelings and passions? Is this whole culture of delicacy, of the small and the pure, perhaps obeying a process of distancing things from reality and idealization? Is what is really happening actually a change in the opposite direction? Does this oh-so-subtle control of natural impulses perhaps indicate repressed anguish, hidden by the official and ideological explanation of love?

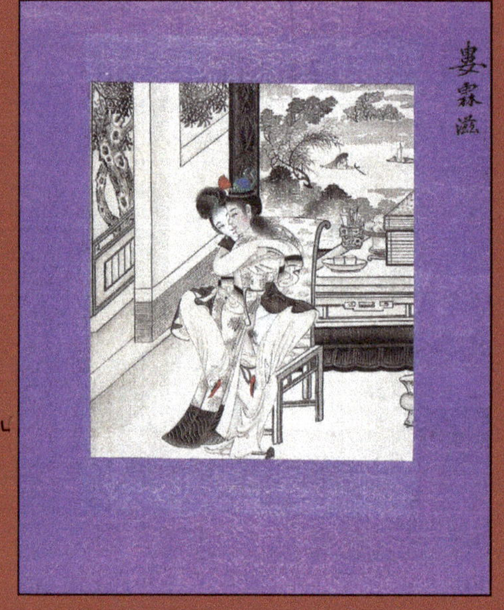

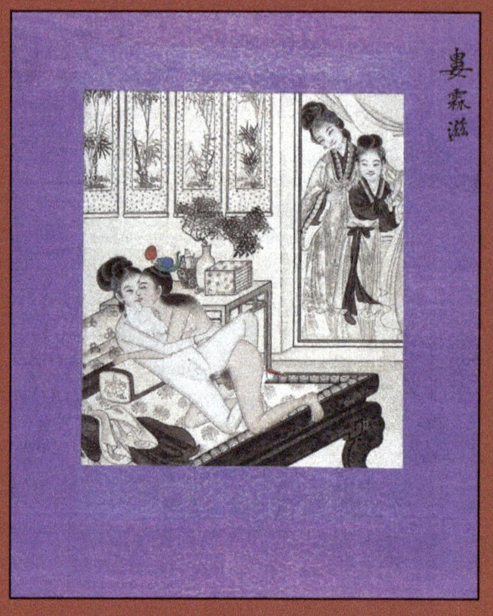

For a man to avoid having an orgasm is clearly, in this day and age, a very reasonable method of birth control: but when this practice is advocated because of the loss of vital energies, one suspects quite another motivation. Is there not here a fear of orgasm, in the form of a fear of the oneiric dilution of one's self?

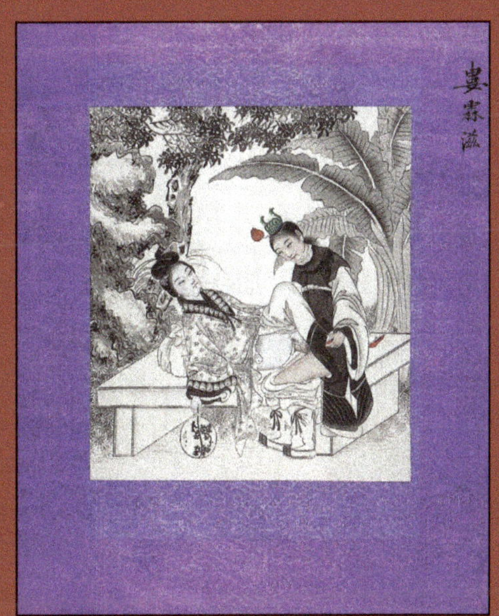

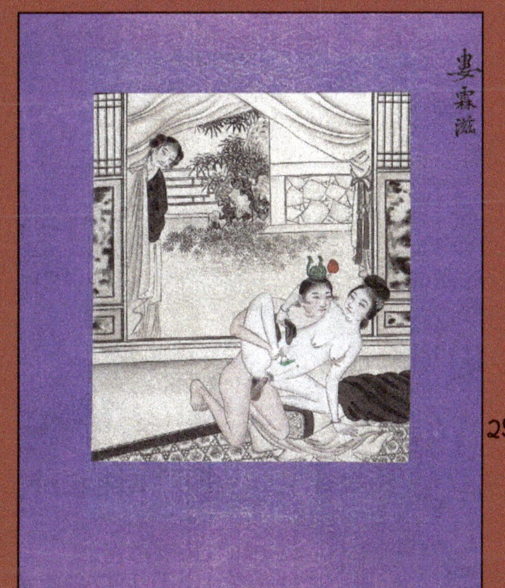

Orgasm, indeed, means 'little death', because during an orgasm for a moment the barriers of the individual are broken down. To flee death: would that not mean, in this male-centred sexuality, fleeing union with a woman? Does the fear of death really mean a fear of women's power? Chastity can only be dangerous, but seeing the loss of sperm as the loss of the very substance of life is no less so.

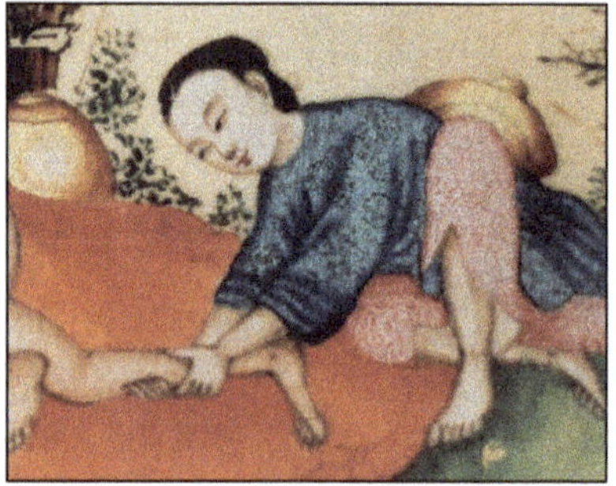

If a young man neglects his sexual life, he will be haunted by phantoms which will rear up in his dreams in the form of seductive young women. If he gives in to them, they will suck out his vital energy. It is exactly on this point that Chinese and European traditions meet. In this dream, it is the unconscious which is reclaiming its rights. Thus, regular sexual relations are recommended.

In this sense, Chinese sexuality seems to be held hostage between two distinct fears: on the one side, there is the fear of losing one's vital energy because of sexual abstention, and on the other is the fear of losing one's vital energy by ejaculating.

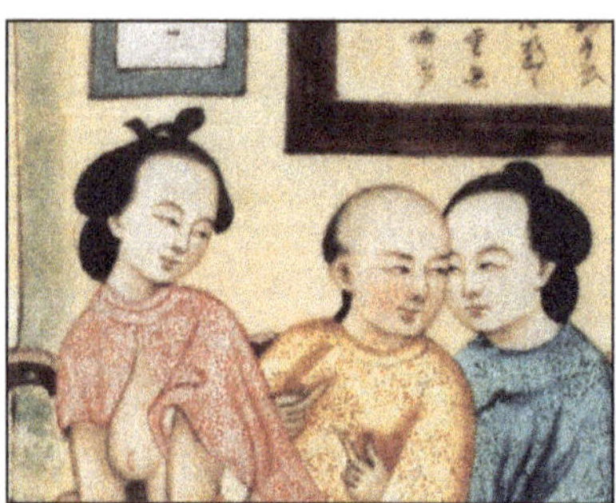

Sharing as we all do the human condition, that is, having all been born from a mother and a father who, in one way or another, have to come to terms with the Oedipus complex, sexuality can only consist, even in China, of a mixture of pleasure and pain. It is exactly these elements that one must seek behind these endless affirmations of eternal harmony.

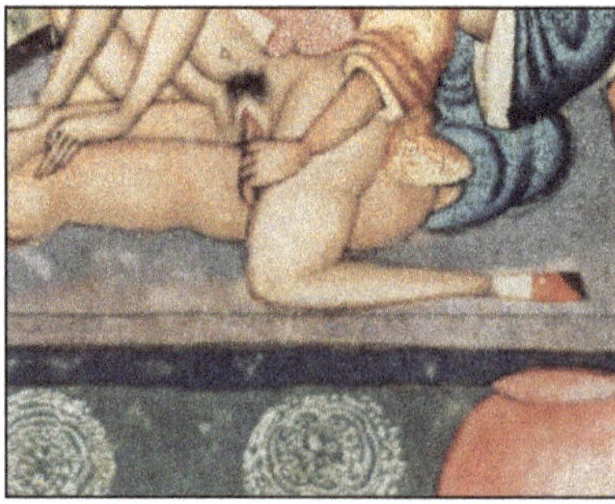

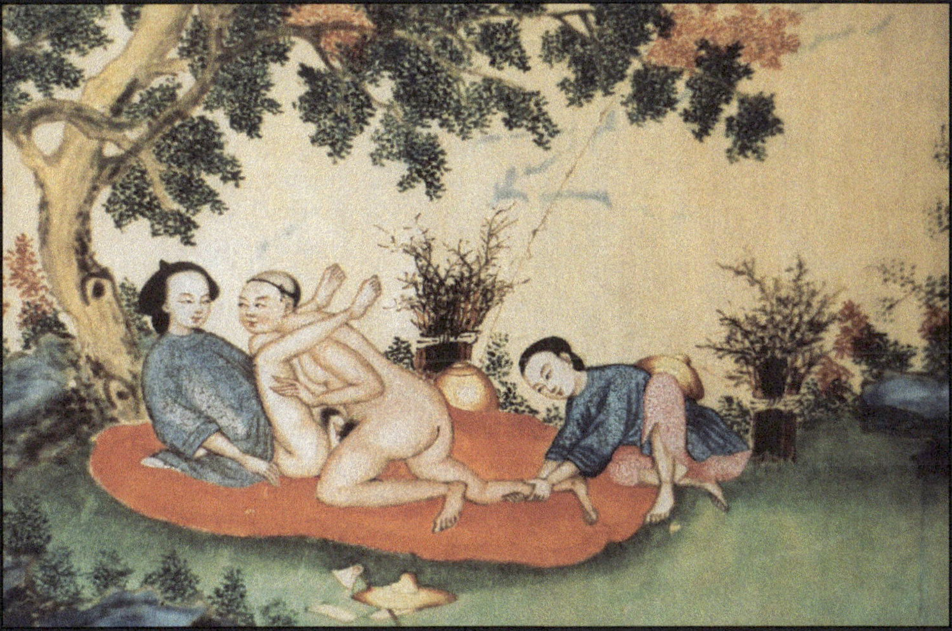

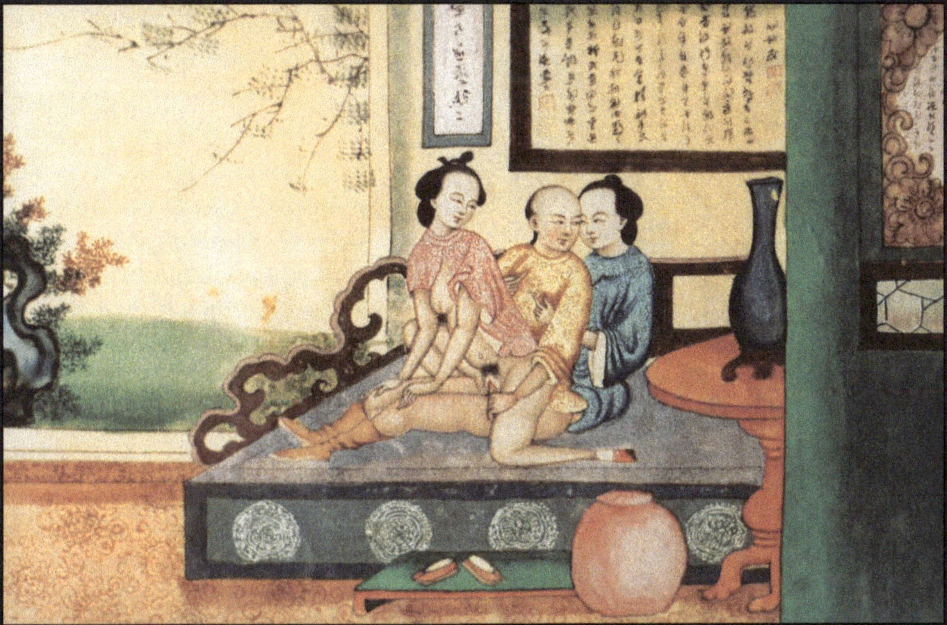

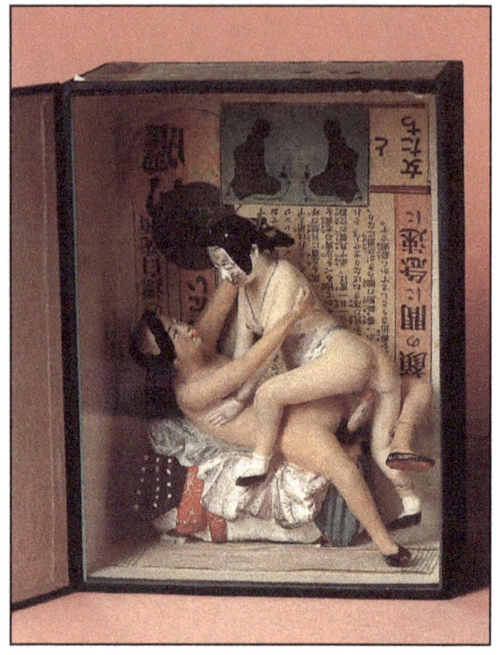

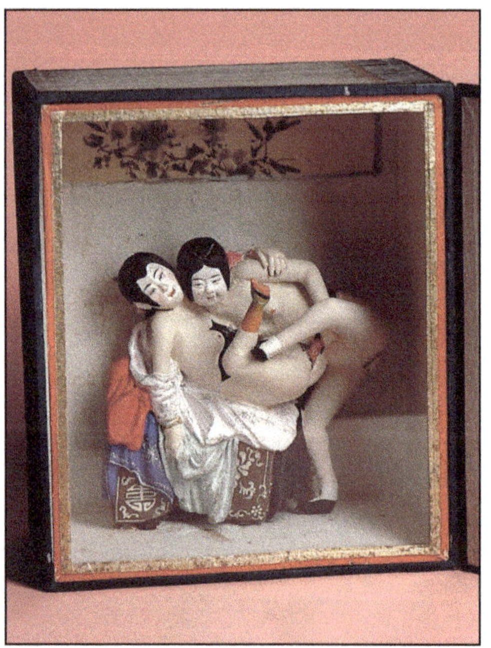

What, for example, is the significance of that fact that, in hundreds and hundreds of depictions of the sexual act, which claim to offer a complete guide to all conceivable sexual positions, I have only found two or three images of cunnilingus? Was this position forbidden? In 1,000 erotic images, only three represent this theme. Isn't that strange?

Likewise, another theme can give us an insight into repressed fears:

In all the images that we have seen, women wear their shoes, even if they are naked. Unshod feet are never shown. For the Chinese, these feet, enclosed in their embroidered shoes, represented the most sublime erotic quality, and small feet exerted a very specific charm over men which we find difficult to understand today. During the Ming period, the custom of foot-binding developed rapidly. Concubines, courtesans, and also simple, mainly peasant women, had their feet broken in childhood and then had them bound for the rest of their lives. Any refusal of this custom was considered shameful. When in 1644 an attempt was made to abolish the custom, the women of Manchuria practically revolted. Indeed, this sign of nobility was held particularly dear among the poorest elements of the population. The bound foot represented at the same time the most powerful taboo: if a woman allowed her foot to be touched without resisting too strongly, one could hope for anything from her.

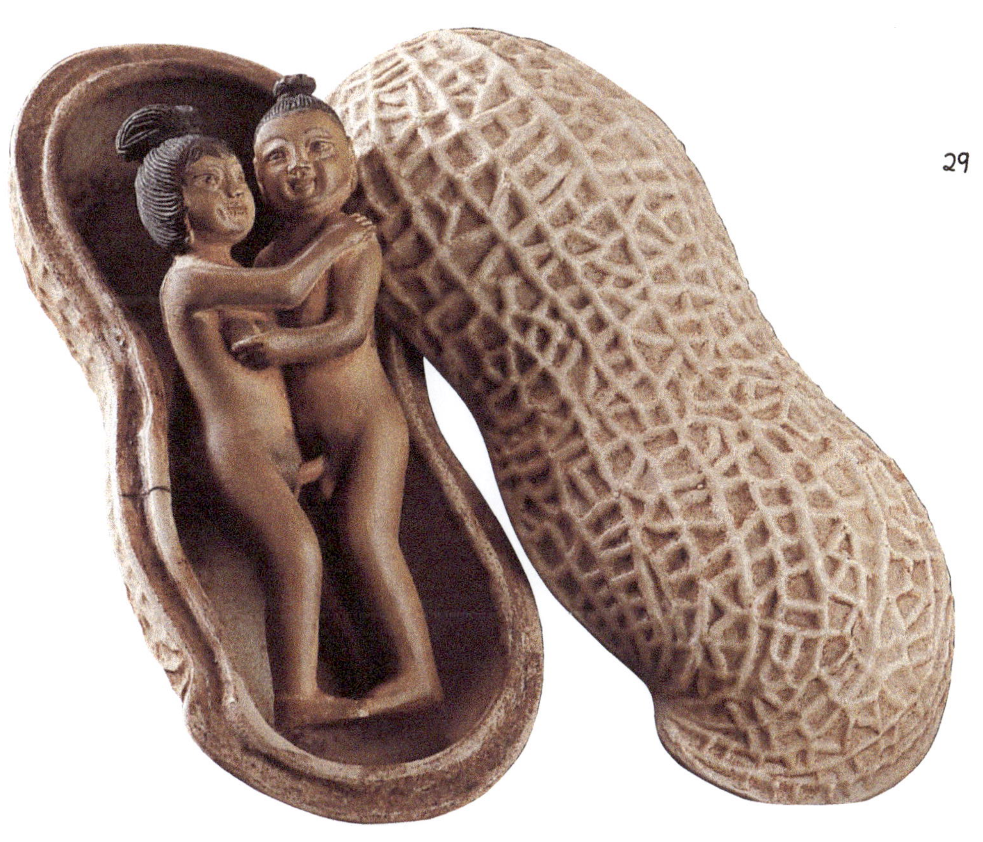

29

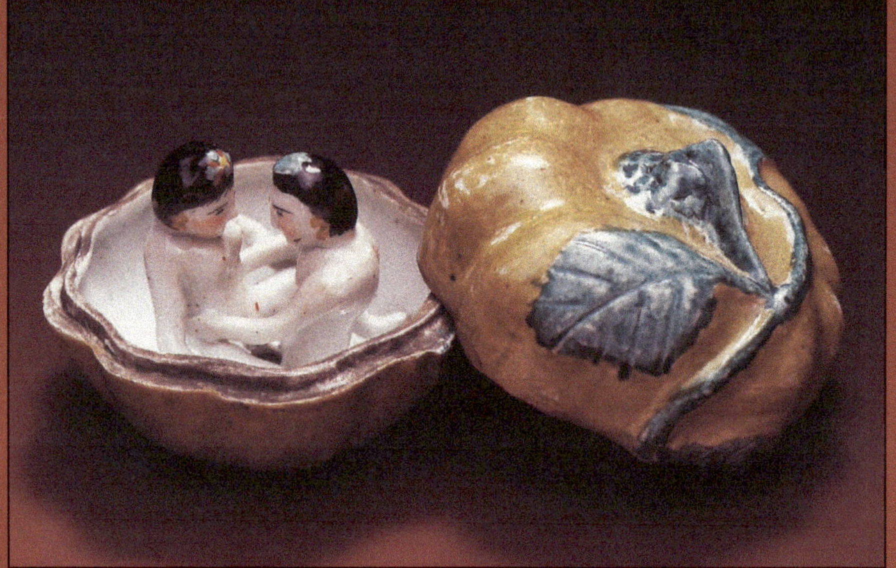

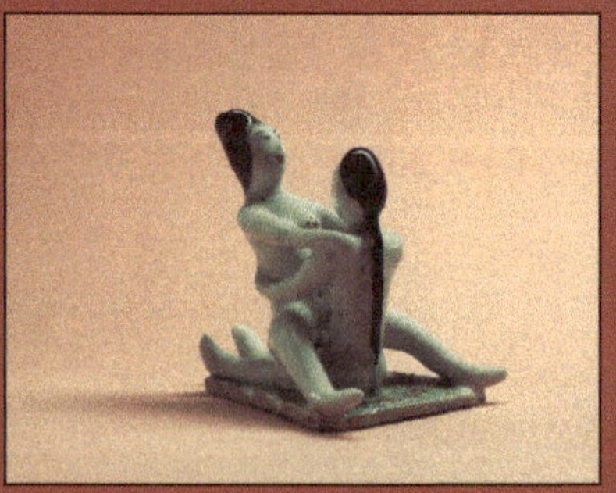

30

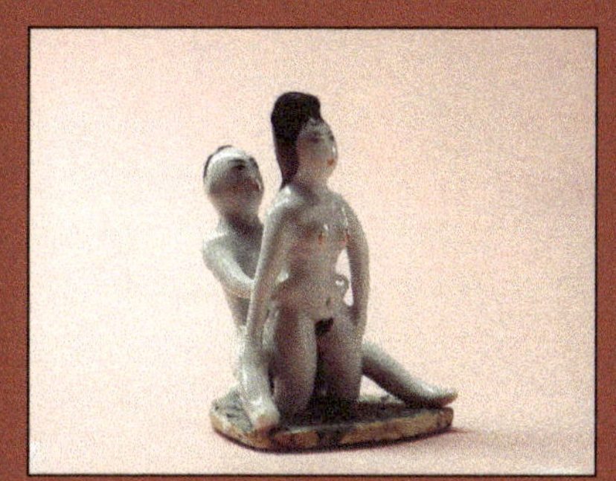

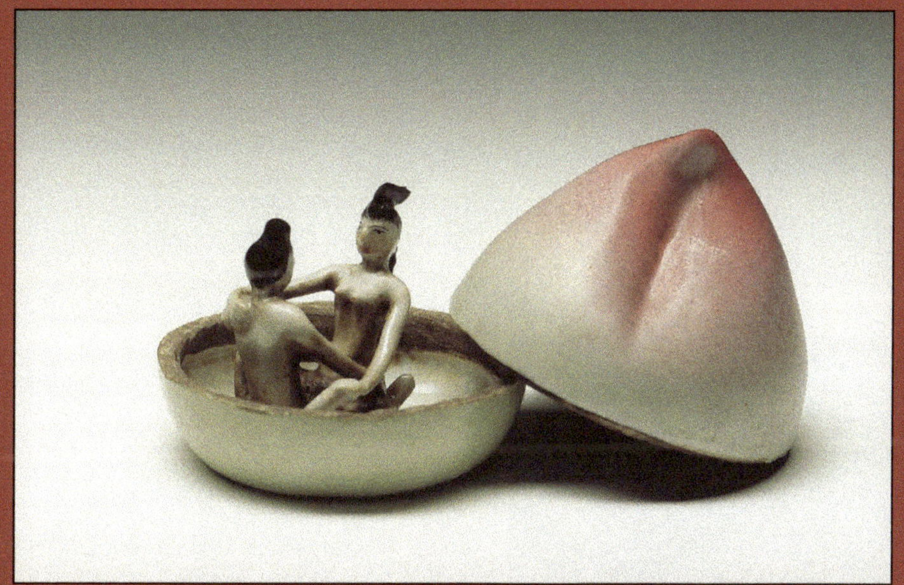

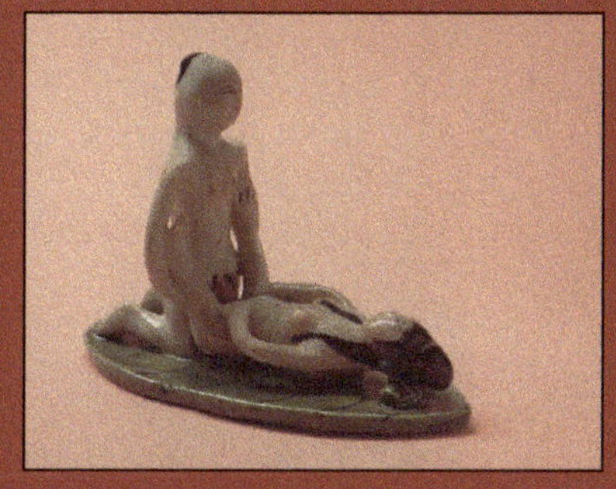

32

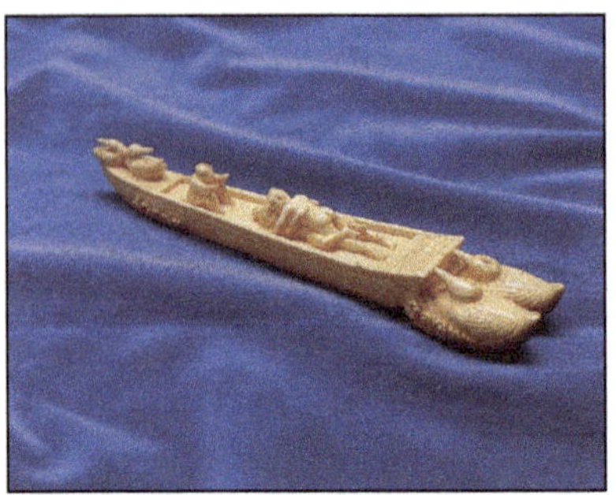

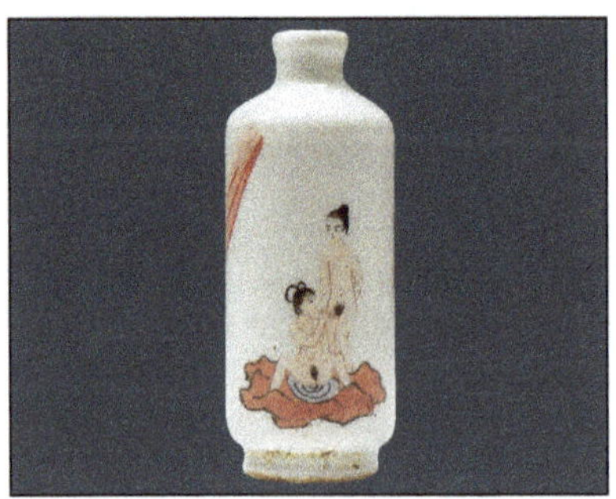

This custom was finally abolished by Mao Tse-Tung in 1949.

Some authors have posited the theory that this 'walk of the golden lotuses' tightened the vaginal muscles, but there is no medical proof to sustain the idea.

Etiemble suggests that the bound feet of Chinese women 'has nothing to do with what was and still is the essence of Chinese eroticism: the theory of Yin and Yang, the coitus reservatus, the respect for the partner's orgasm and the naturalness of feelings.'

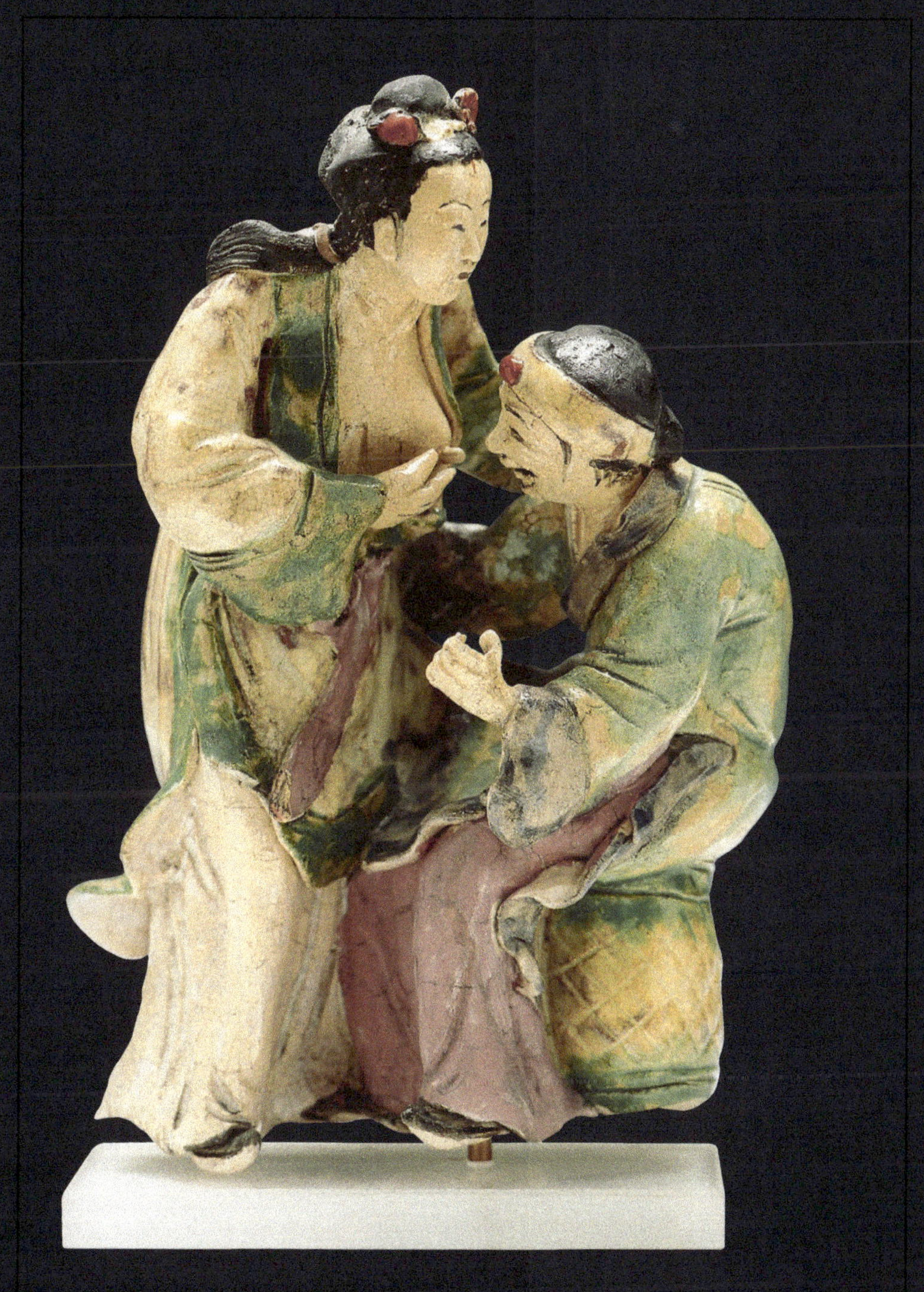

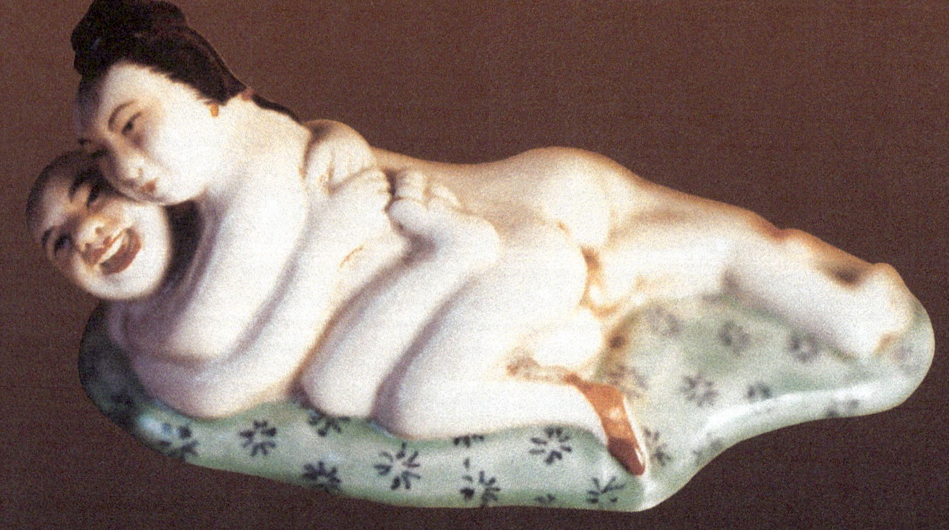

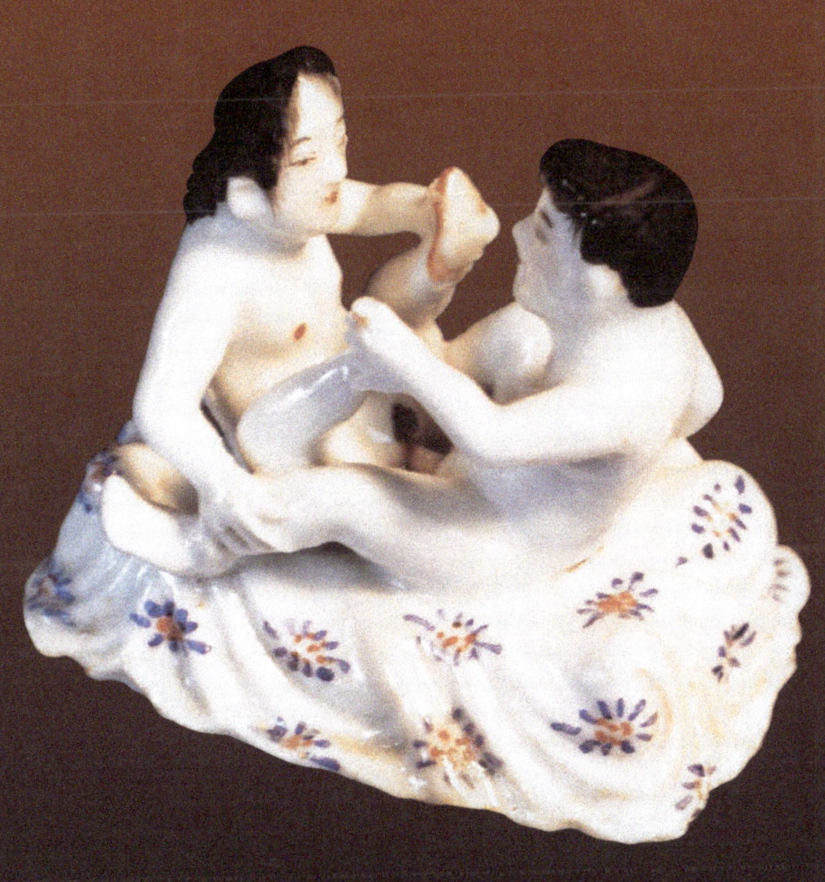

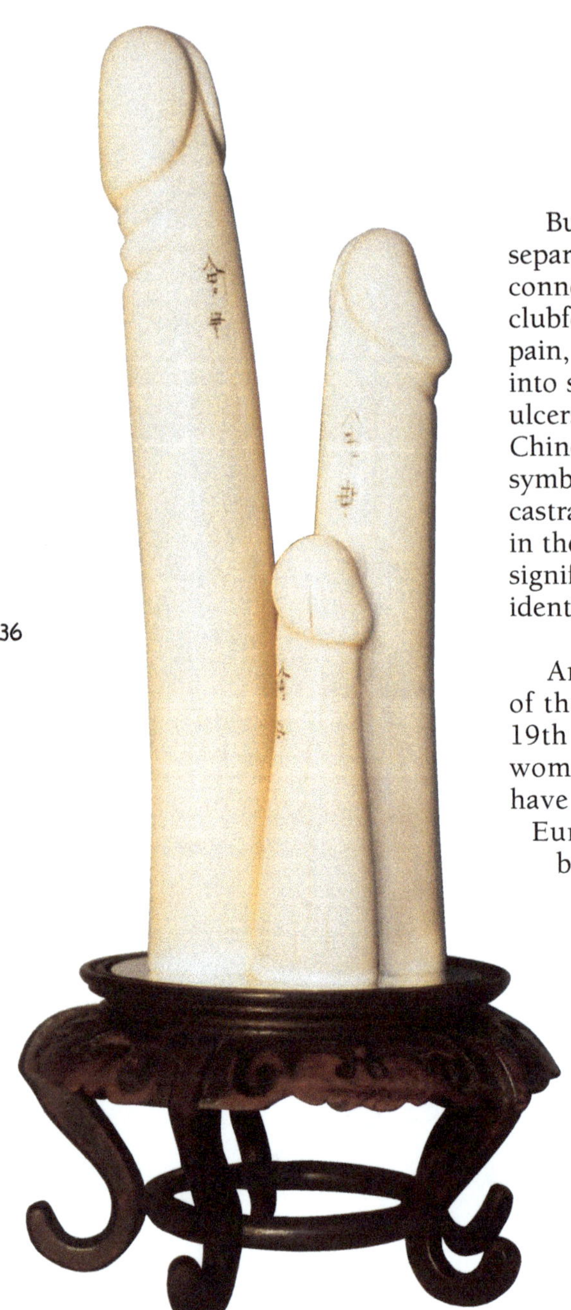

But perhaps we are seeking to separate things that are in fact connected. If one thinks about it - a clubfoot acquired through appalling pain, flattened ankles which sink into stockings filled with painful ulcers: this has nothing to do with Chinese eroticism. Is it not a symbolic castration of woman? A castration which found redress only in the woman's toe, the phallic significance of which was swiftly identified?

And what about the treatment of the female body during the 19th century? Does trussing women up in wired corsets not have some connection with European eroticism? The female body, sadistically laced up and suffocated by handcuffs and belts: is that not a fundamental indication of man's primal fear of woman?

36

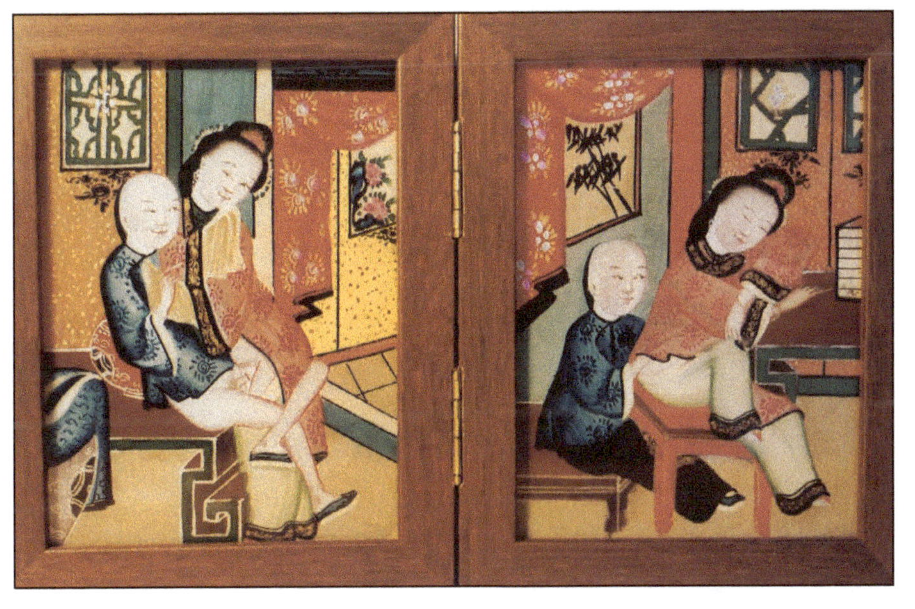

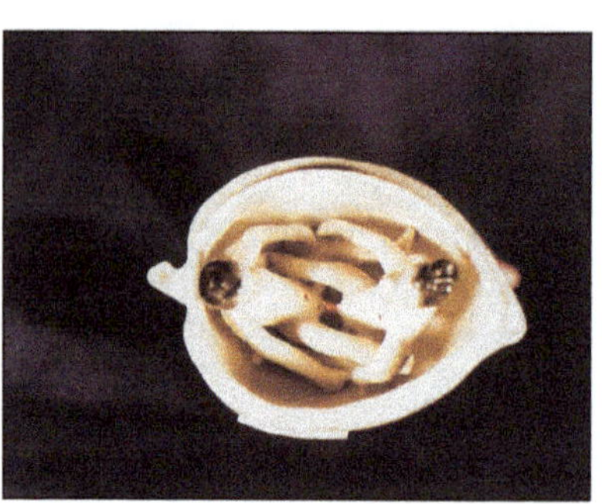

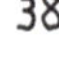
38

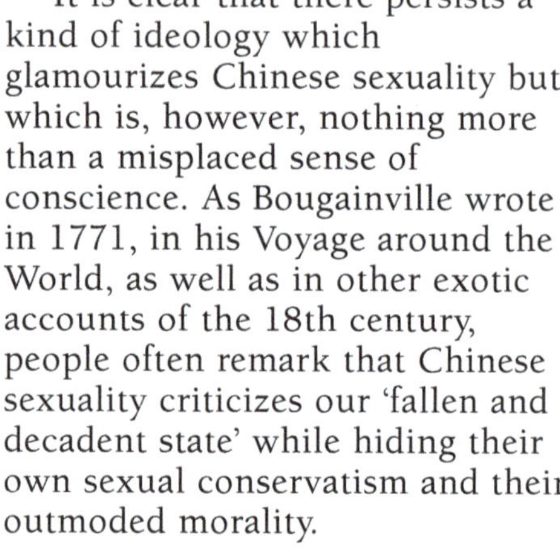

It is clear that there persists a kind of ideology which glamourizes Chinese sexuality but which is, however, nothing more than a misplaced sense of conscience. As Bougainville wrote in 1771, in his Voyage around the World, as well as in other exotic accounts of the 18th century, people often remark that Chinese sexuality criticizes our 'fallen and decadent state' while hiding their own sexual conservatism and their outmoded morality.

Perhaps I too am nothing more than a desperately decadent European who will never be able to find the path to the noble art that is love.

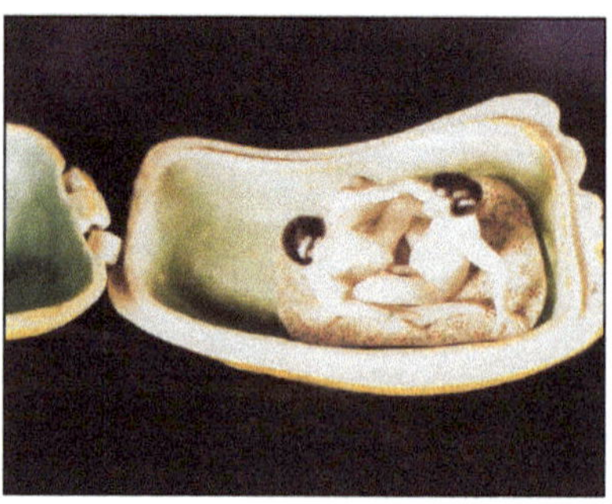

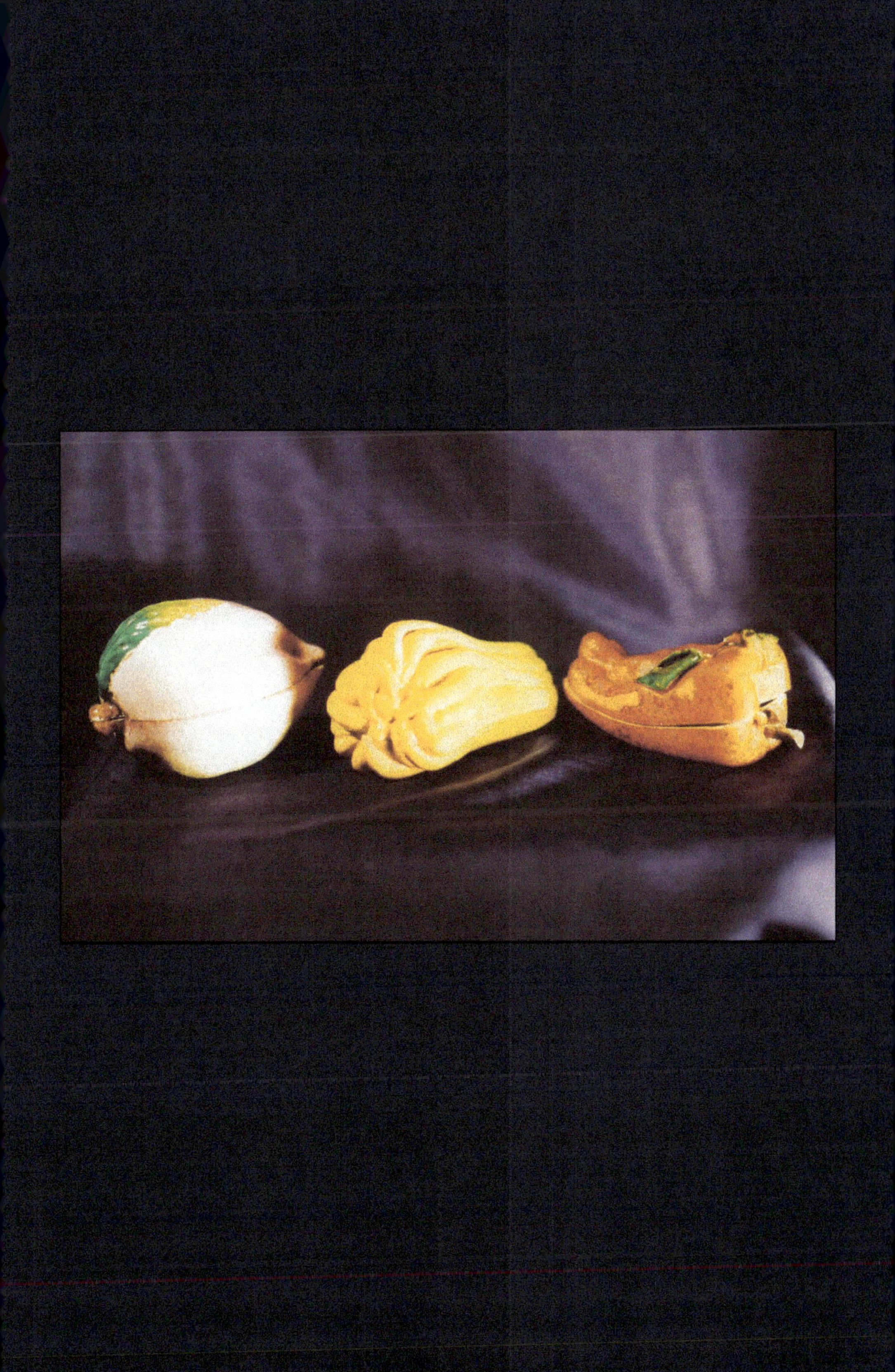

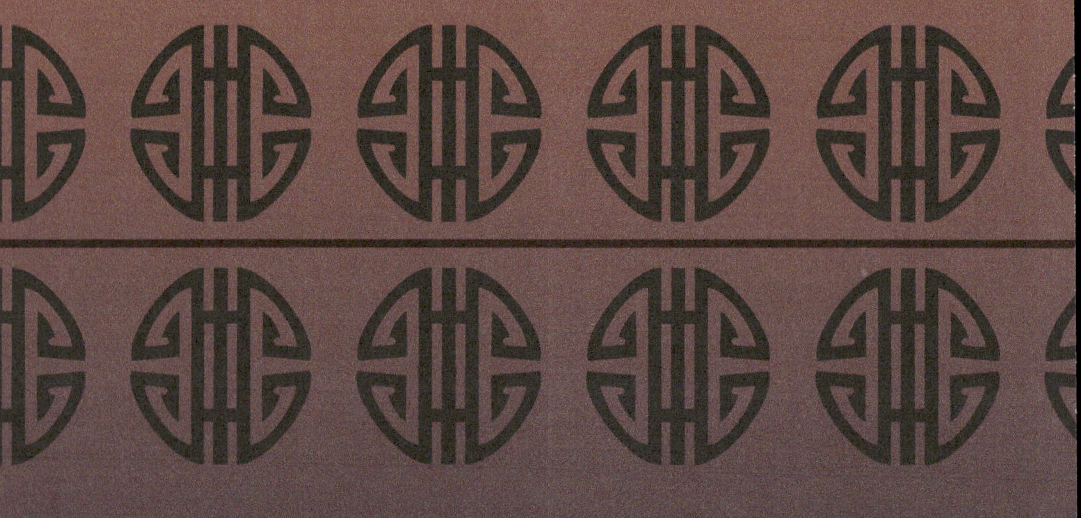

JAPANESE EROTIC

ENGRAVINGS

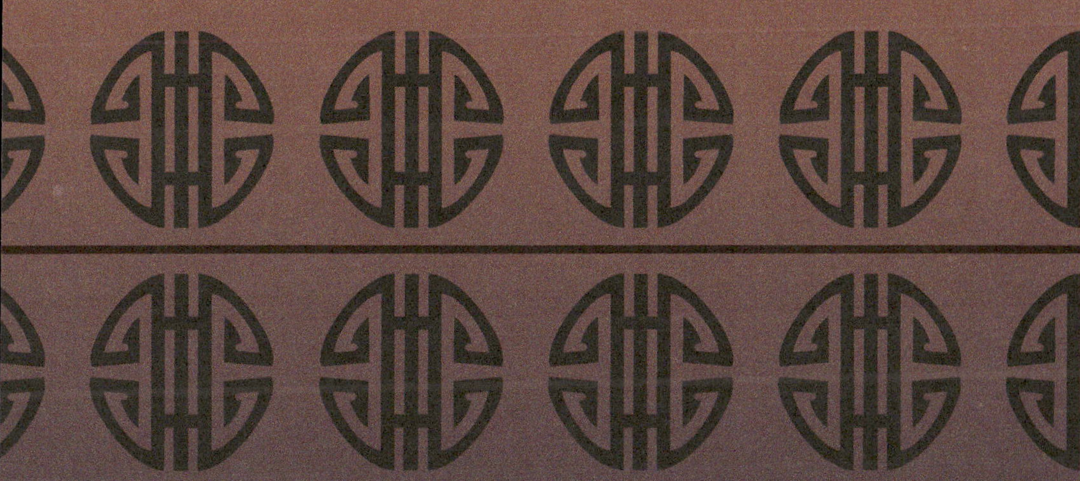

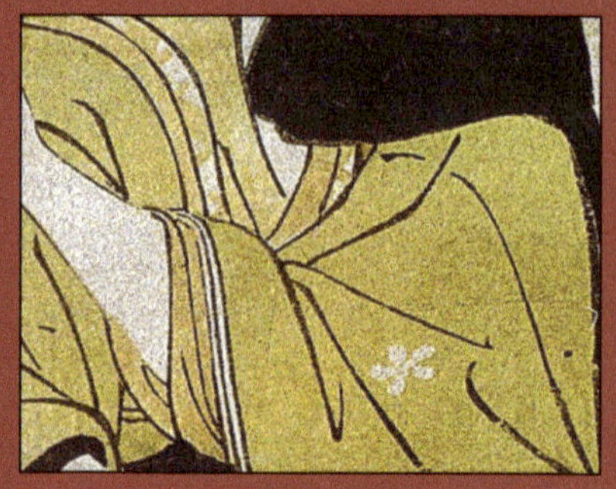

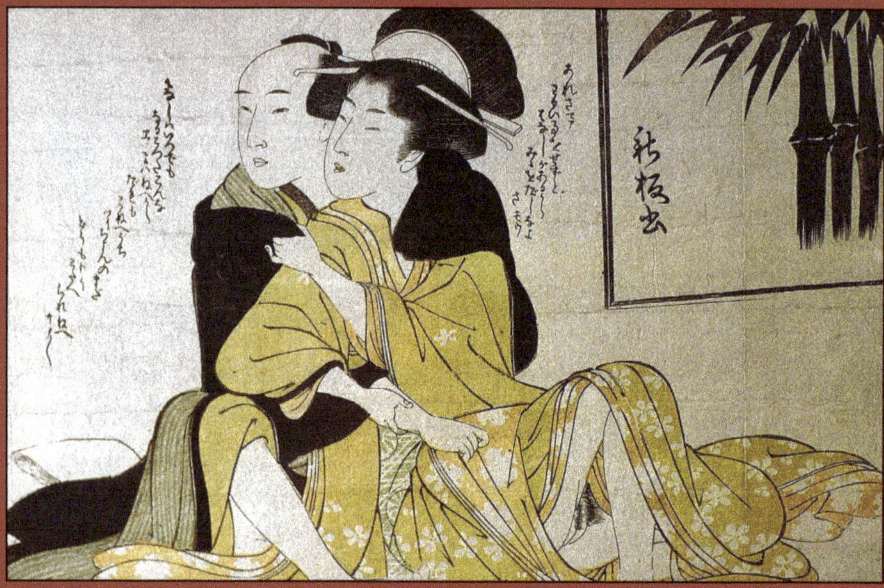

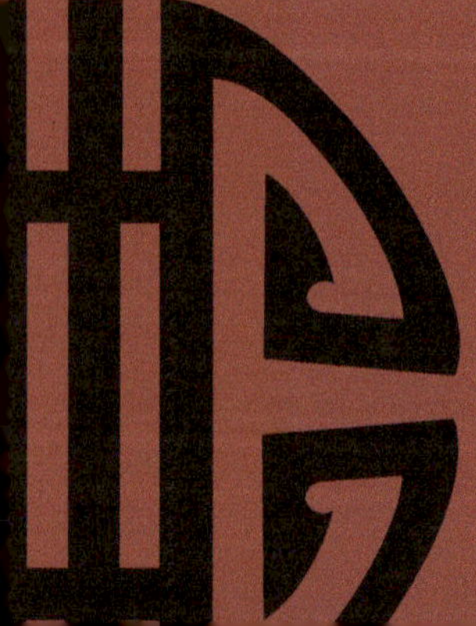

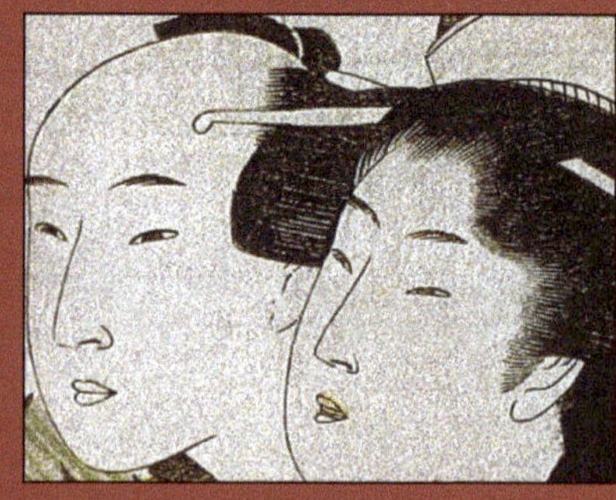

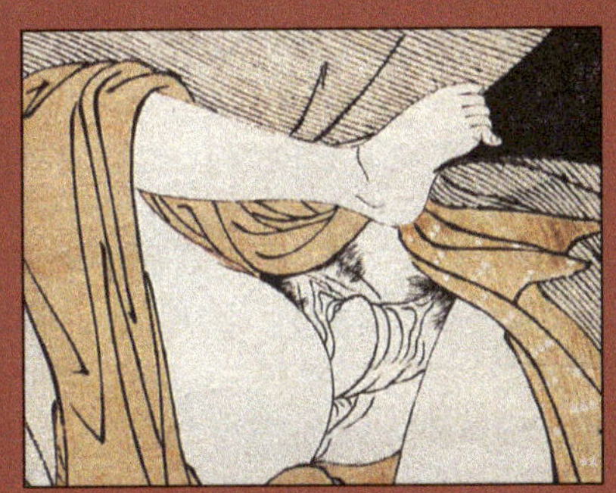

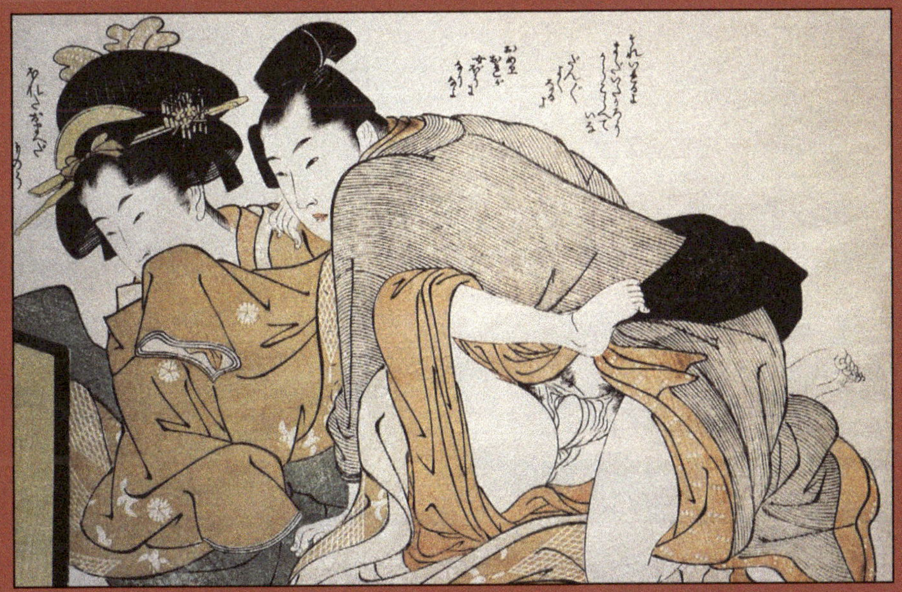

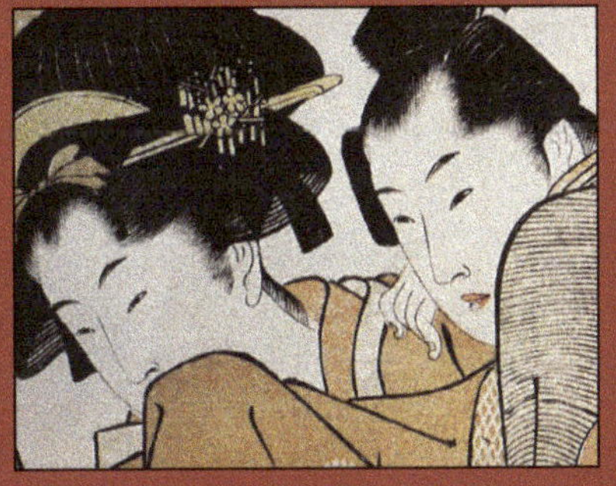

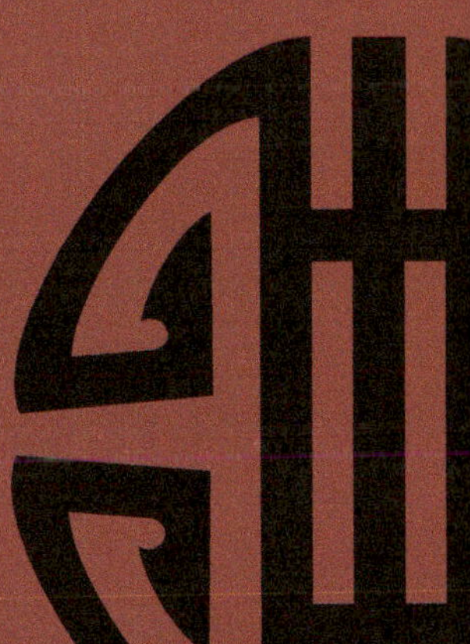

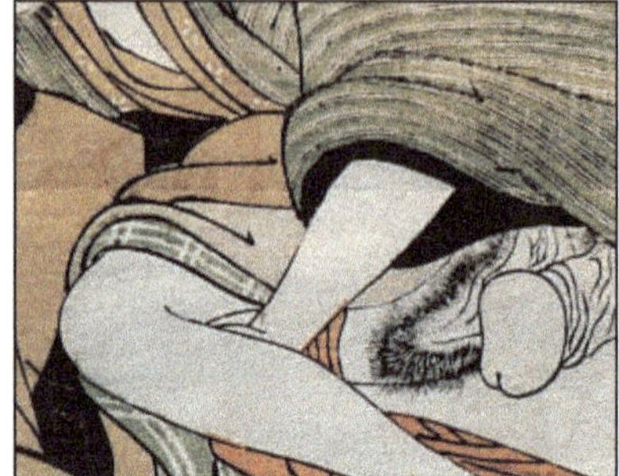

Between the sublime and the grotesque

Japanese erotic engravings

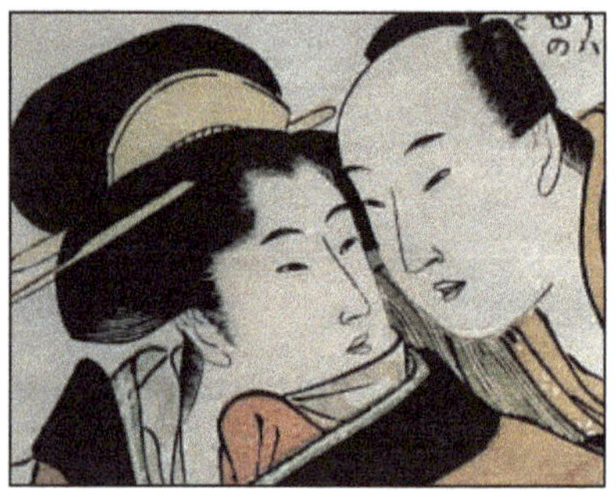

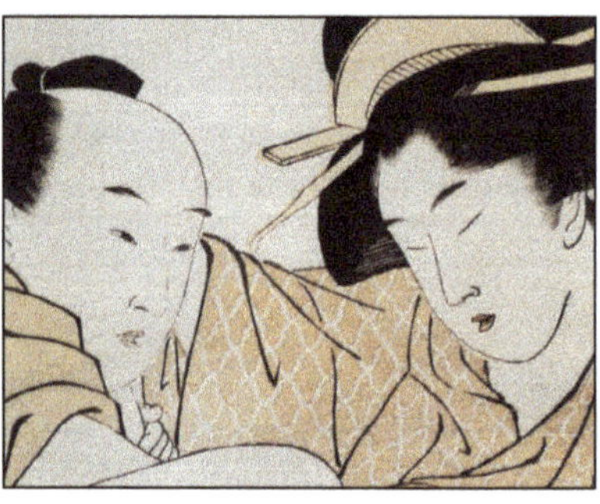

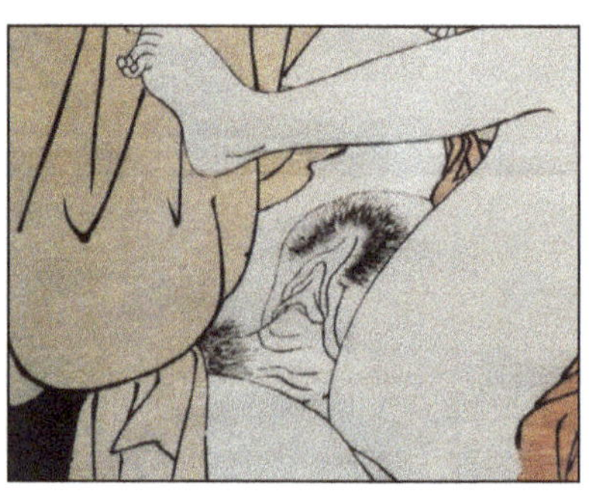

In contrast with classical Japanese art, books of Ukiyo-e woodcarvings show 'images of a changing, ephemeral and perishable world.' We know them under the name shunga, which means 'spring picture.'

The term shunga originally came from Buddhism and is associated with the idea of the painful vanity of all earthly things. Soon, however, its meaning changed as it gradually came to signify the joyful, carefree delights of everyday life, and a playful and unconcerned manner of abandoning oneself to the pleasures of the moment, of letting oneself go with the flow 'like a pumpkin in the currents of a river.' Thus, for the most part, the Ukiyo-e illustrate scenes between courtesans and actors and are set in a world full of pleasure. The shungas allow us a glimpse into a universe where the greedy enjoyment of life is paramount and the pleasures of carnal love play an important role.

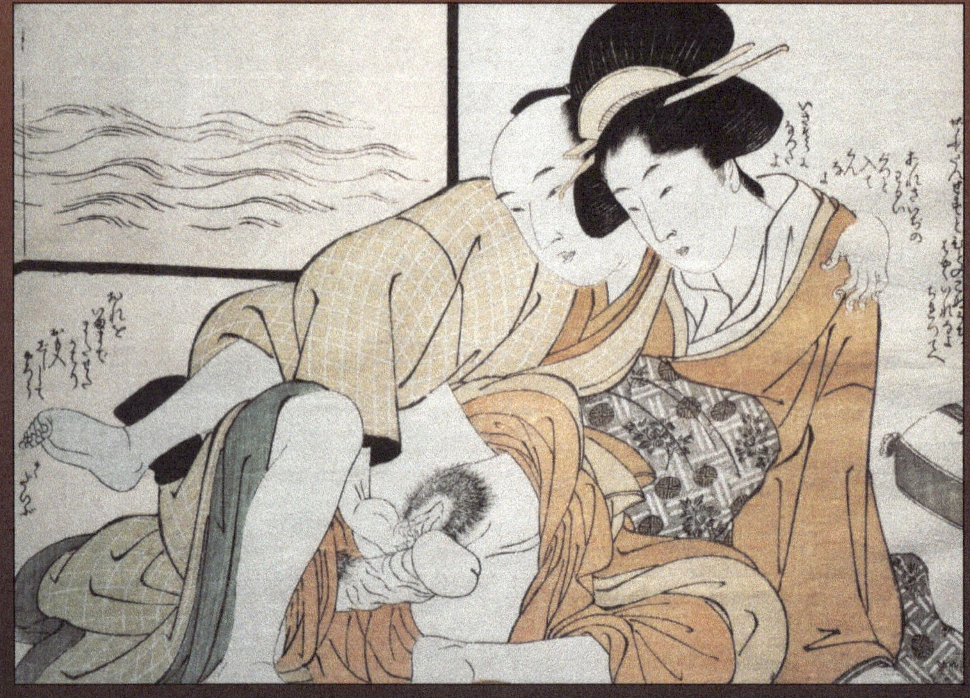

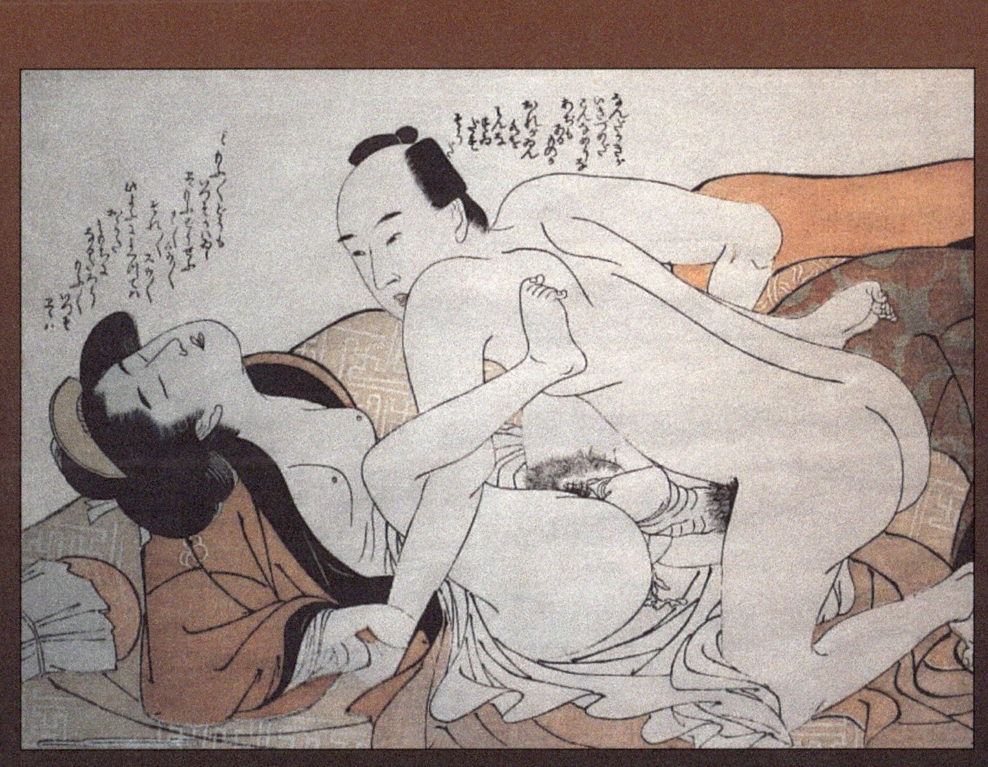

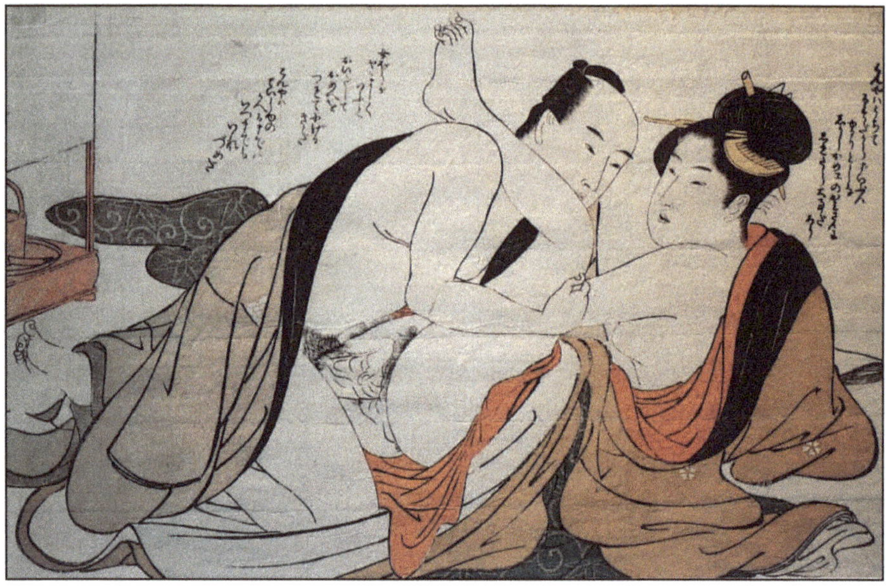

Japanese woodcarving developed over a period of two centuries, between around 1670 to 1870. Utamaro, the undisputed master of colour woodcarving, was active for only three decades of this period, between 1770 and 1800. This also happened to be the golden age of the Ukiyo-e. In his book on Utamaro, Edmond de Goncourt explains the fascination of erotic woodcarving: 'It is really worth studying the erotic paintings of the Japanese, if only because of the amazing pleasure to be had from their drawing, the impetuosity, the natural power of these sexual unions, or because

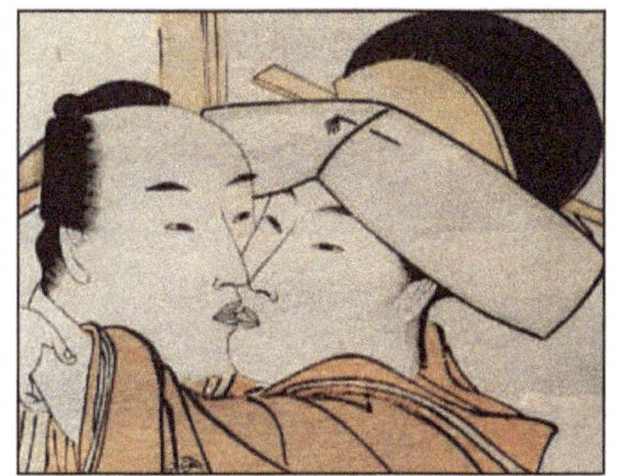

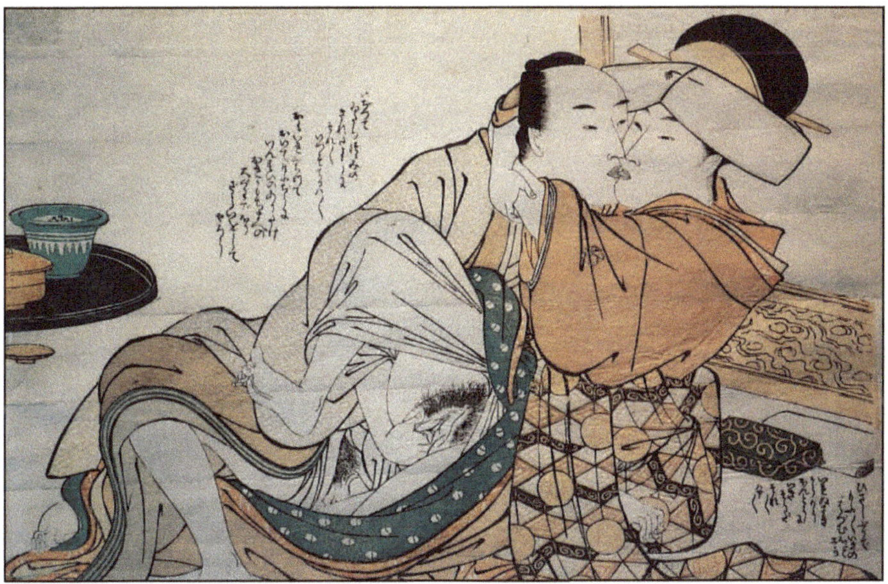

of that uncontrollable desire to make love and push through the paper walls of the next room to do so. What a confusion of bodies, some entangled, some united, what greedy vigour in the arms which both attract and repulse the partner. Feet with curled toes fly through the air, long, deep embraces are exchanged. Eyes closed, eyelids downcast, their faces turned towards the ground, the women look almost as if they have fainted. And finally, look at the force and power with which the man's penis is drawn!'

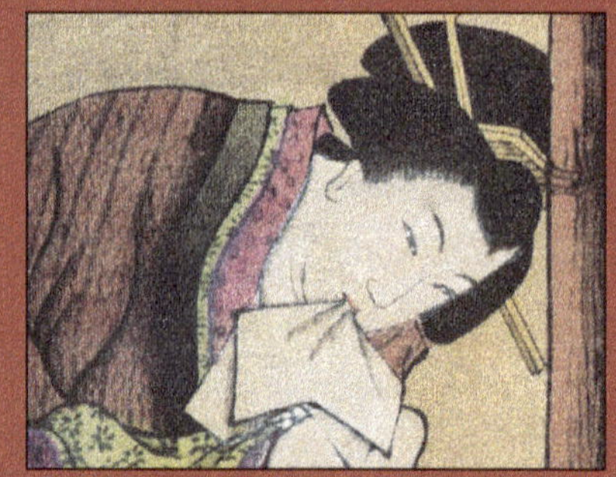

50

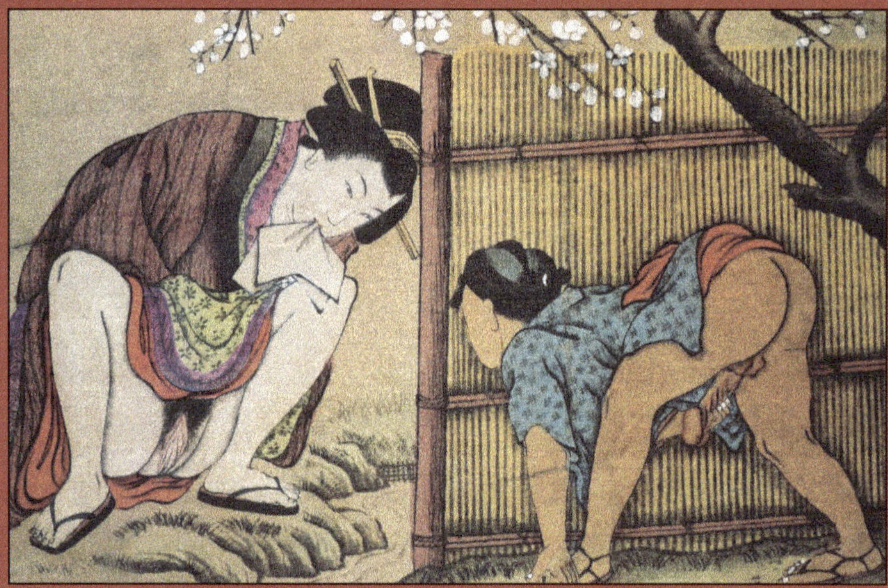

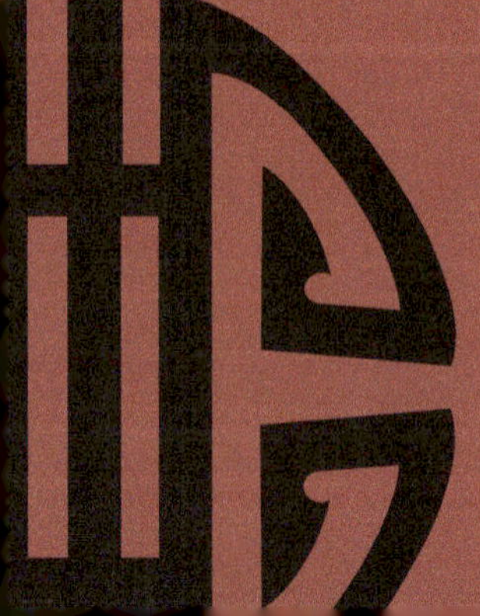

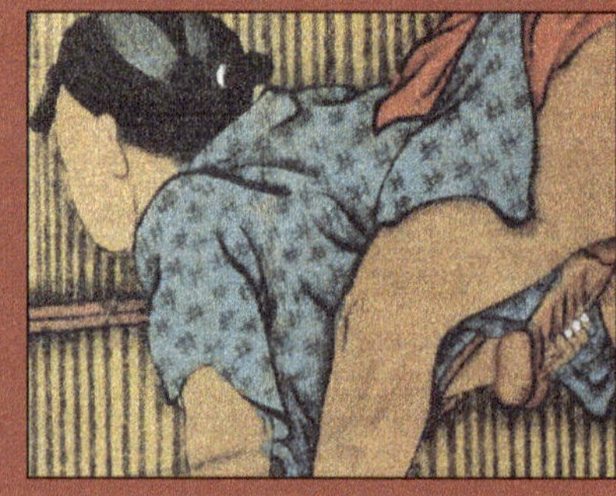

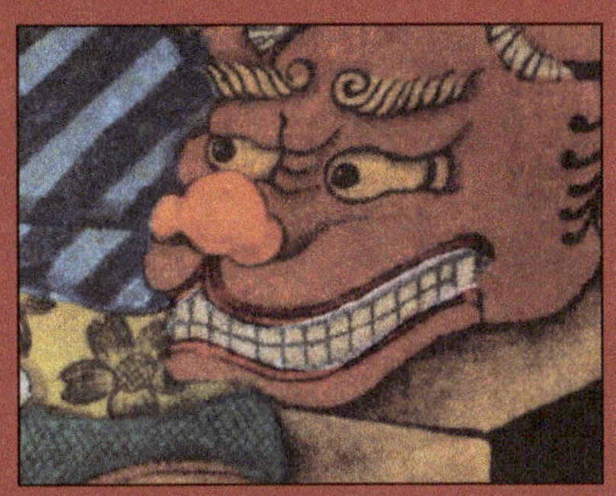

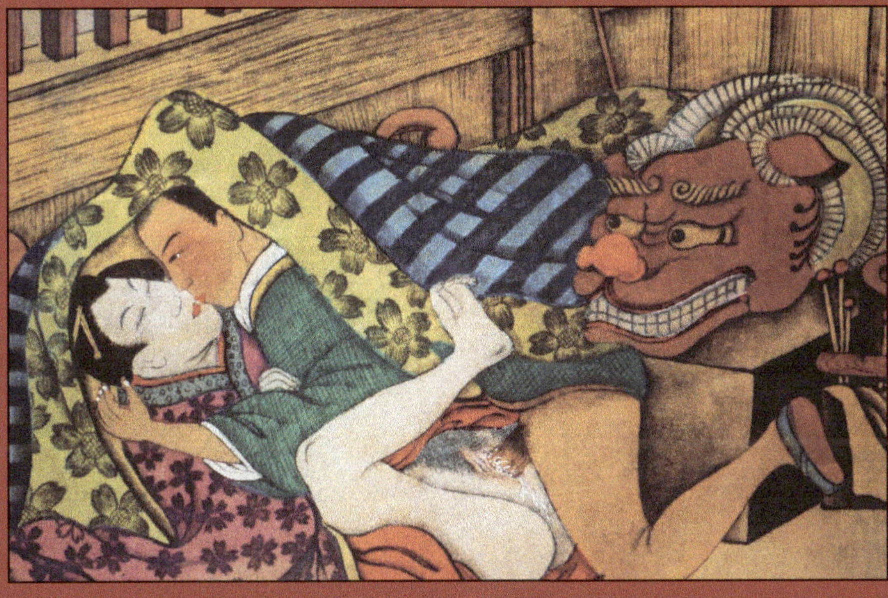

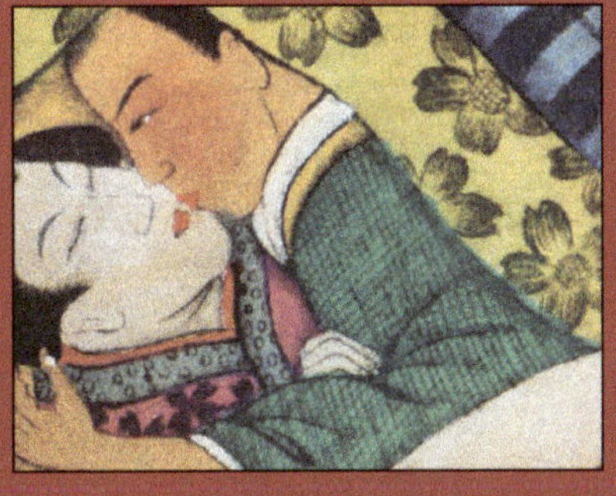

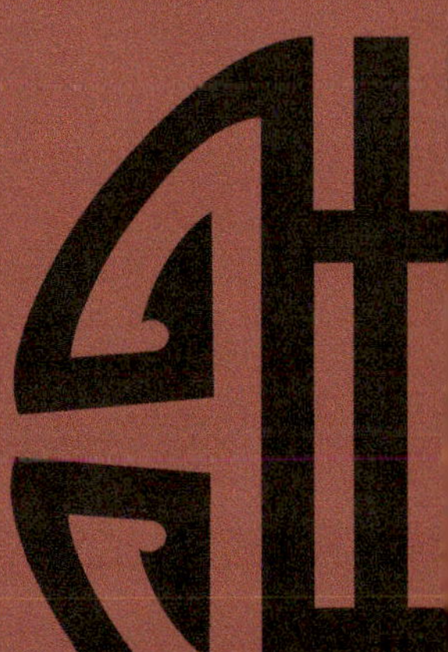

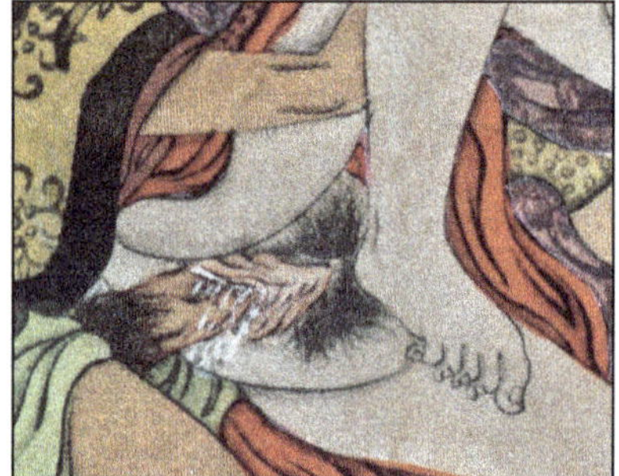

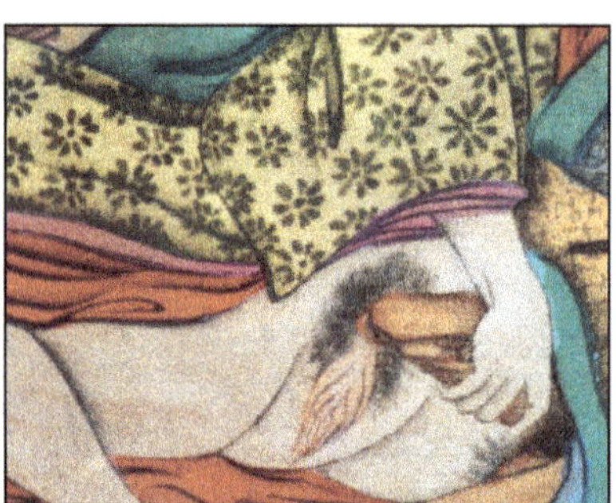

52

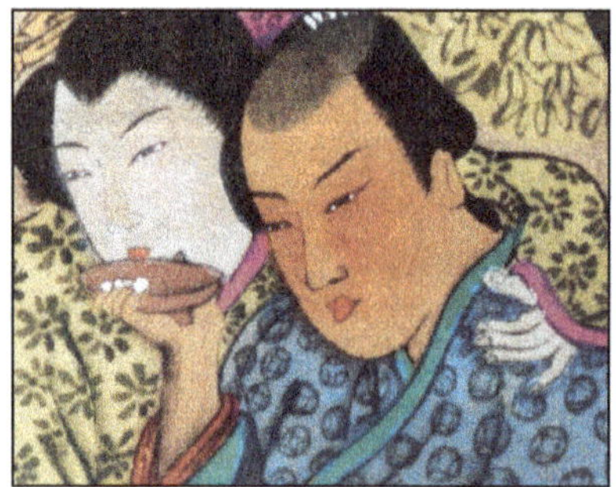

Often, these books and scrolls would form part of a marriage dowry and were supposed to serve as an introduction to the art of lovemaking. In the form of printed or painted scrolls, the shungas thus became family heirlooms. In noble families, they formed part of the sexual education of the young daughter who was destined to become an insatiable lover. They were therefore intended to awaken her sexual imagination but also to bring a particular visual pleasure to the person who contemplated them.

Many of these books were destined for Yoshiwara, the pleasure district in the flourishing city of Edo, in the 17th century. During the Tokugawa period (1600-1853), the rich bourgeois of the big cities who had, during a long period of peace, managed to enrich themselves still further, were enjoying a period of extraordinarily hedonistic pleasure. Districts full of sleazy hotels grew at an astonishing rate until they became the centre of community life. Guides to these 'houses of ill repute' were written, describing in minute detail the charms and defects of the most famous courtesans, not omitting to mention the girls' prices, of course.

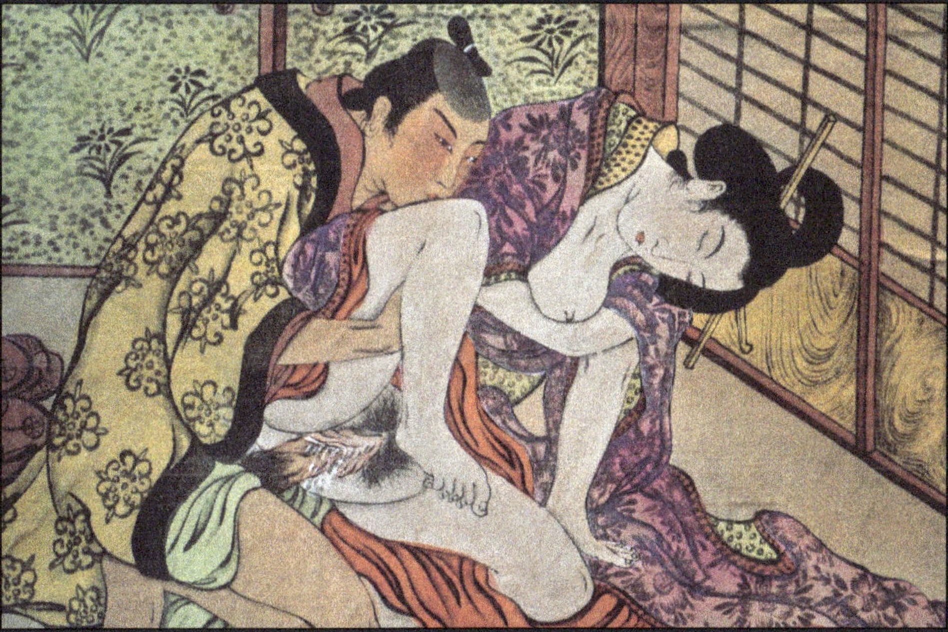

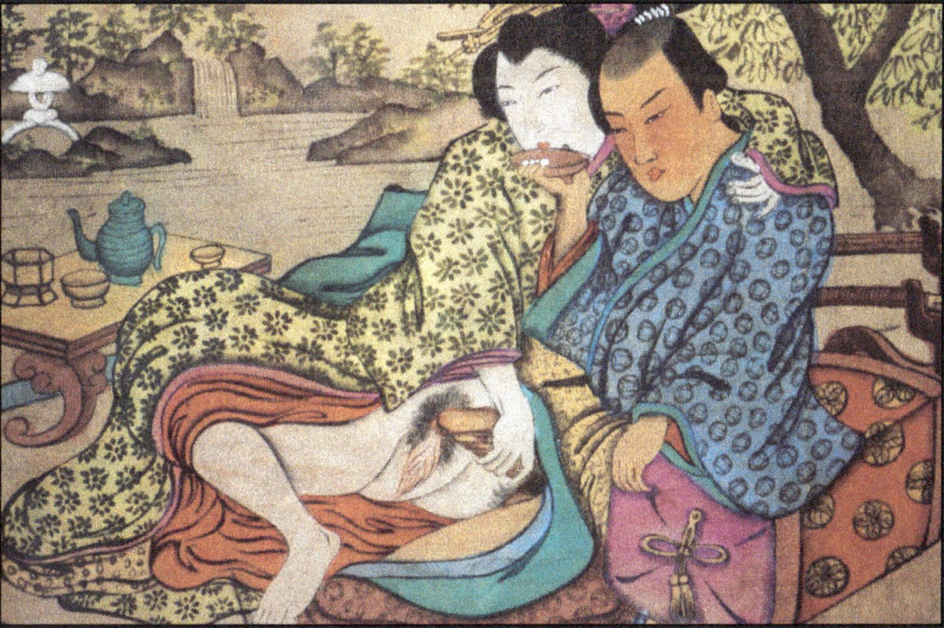

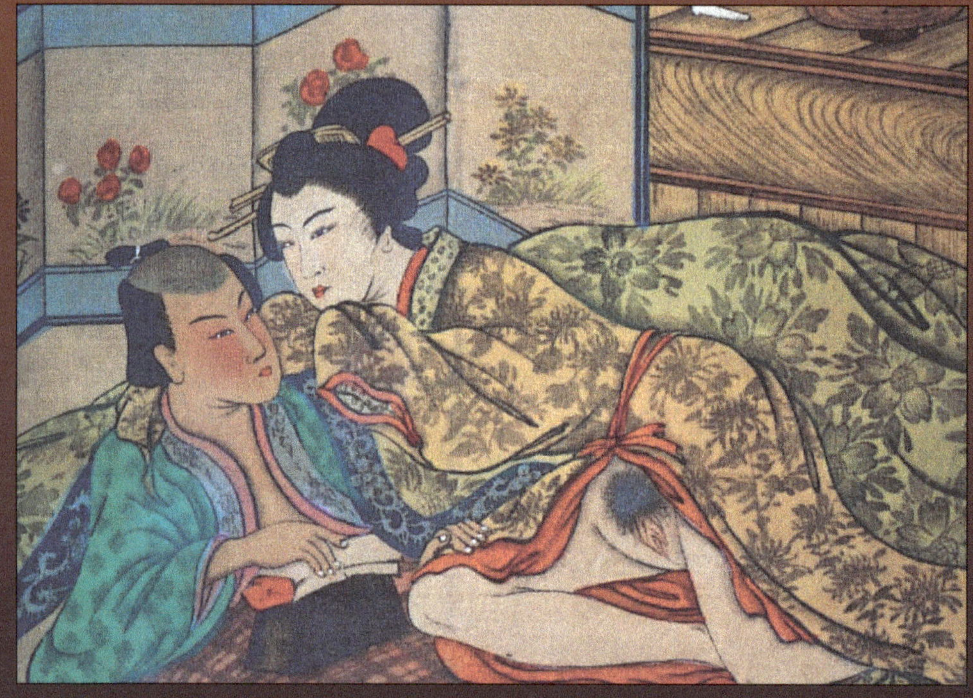

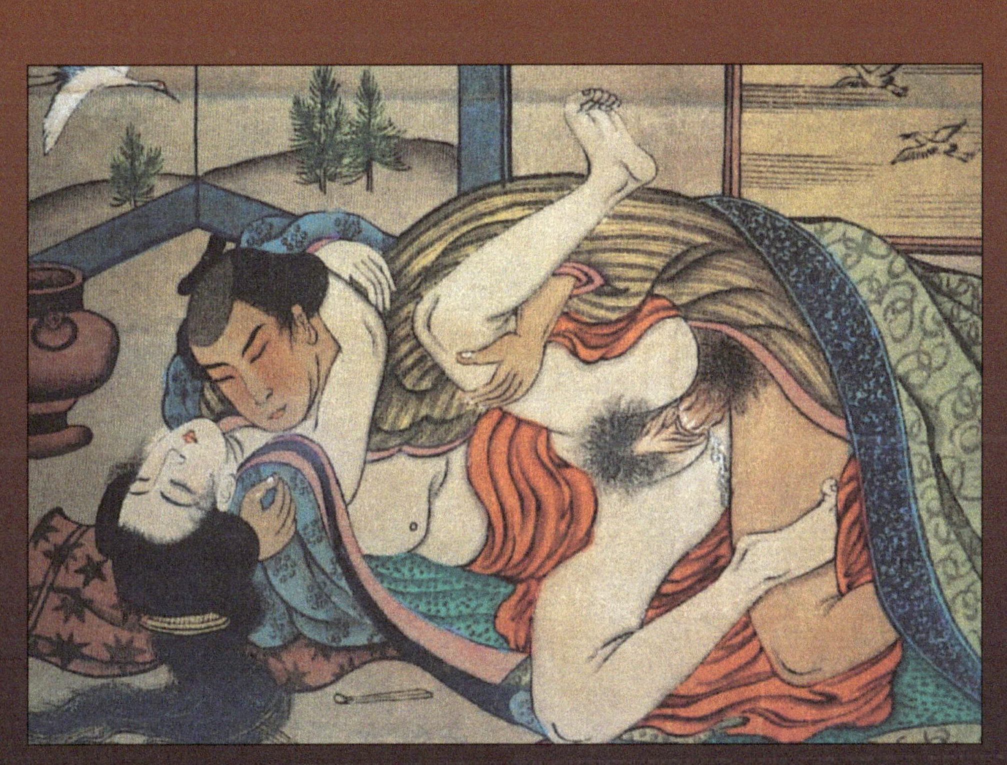

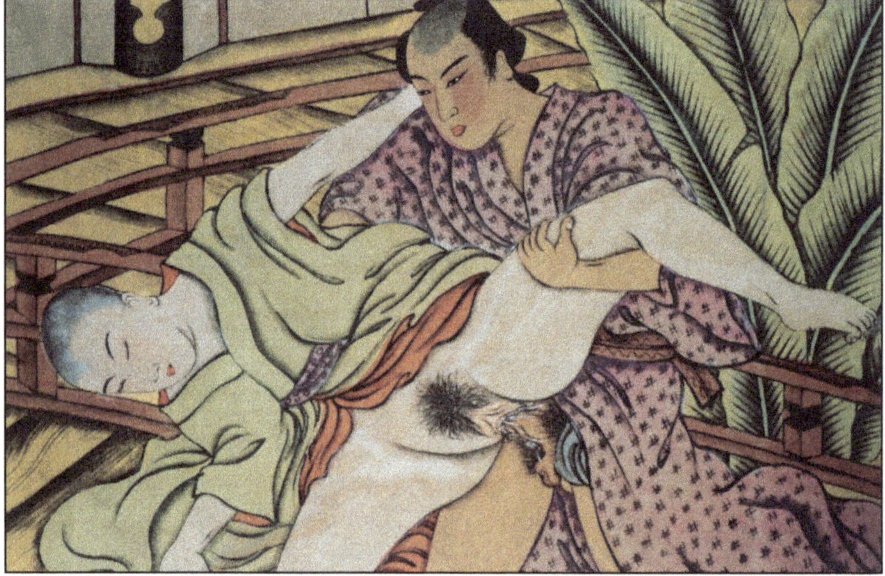

56

These 'love guides' also contained information concerning the women's characters: which of the concubines was particularly clever and innovative, who was loyal and who was sincere. Other books gave lists of intimate details, with advice about how to behave with the women and explaining the sexual practices that were specific to each one. For connoisseurs, there was even information about where one could find rare and unusual pleasures.

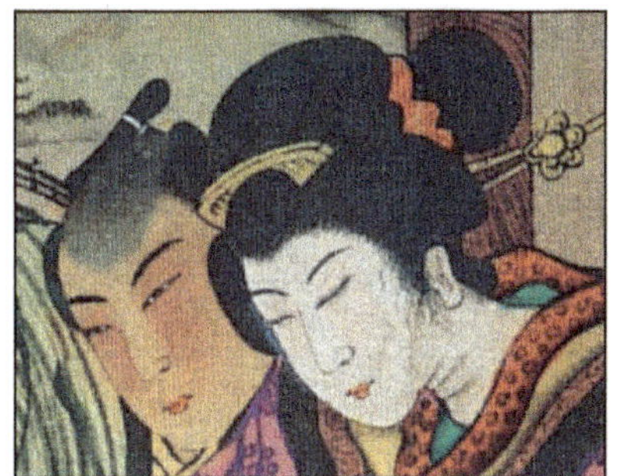

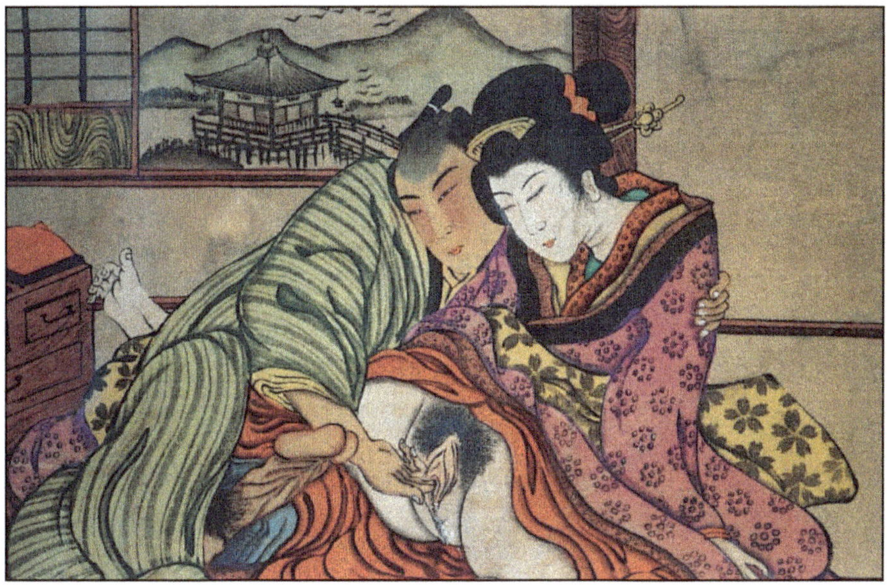

The collector and businessman
Hayashi Tadamasa (1851-1906),
who was one of the first to bring
these precious Japanese
woodcarvings to Paris, owned no
less than two hundred 'guides to
the houses of pleasure,' describing
the life of the courtesans of
Yoshiwara.

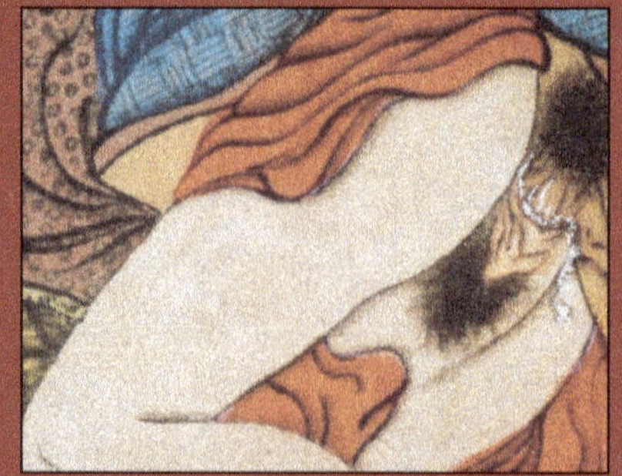

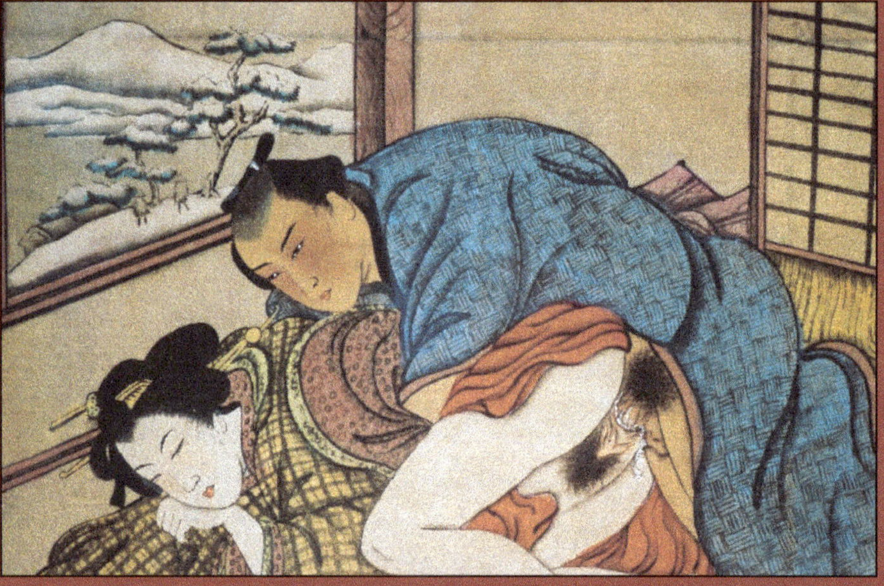

58

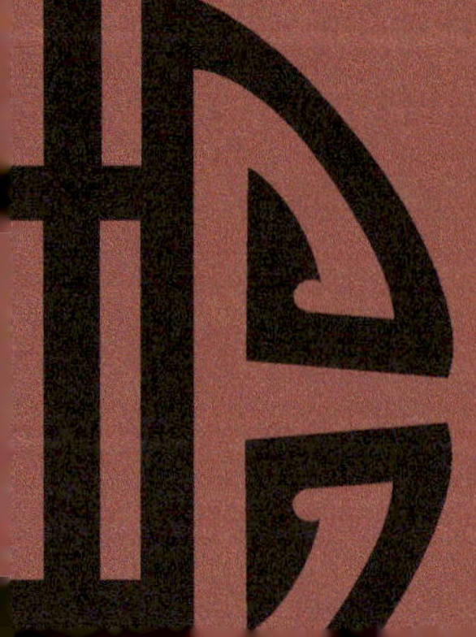

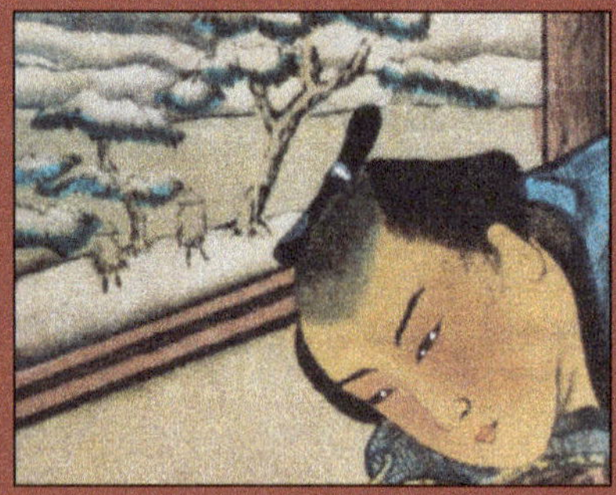

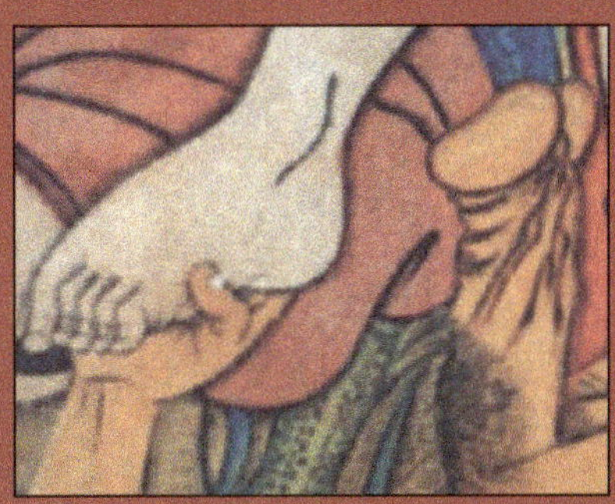

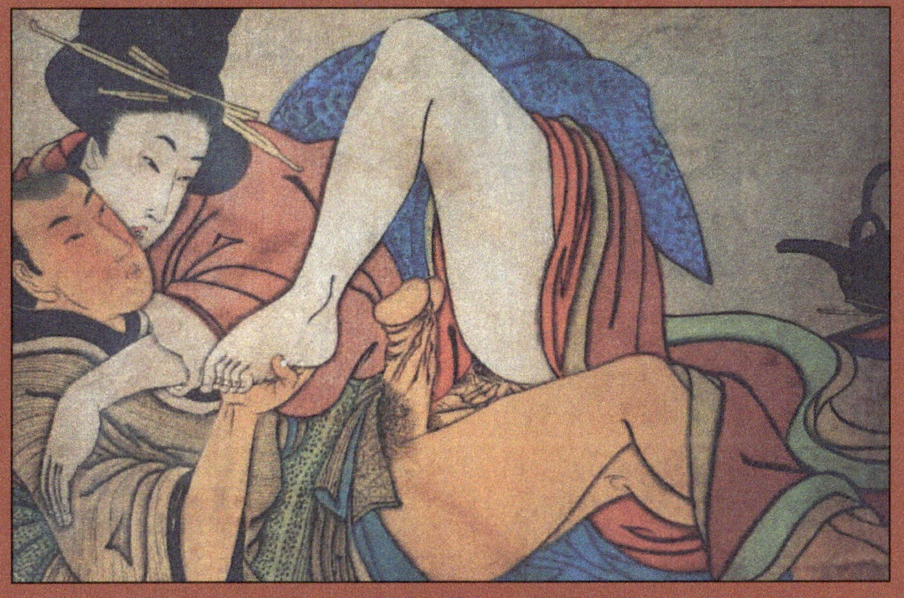

59

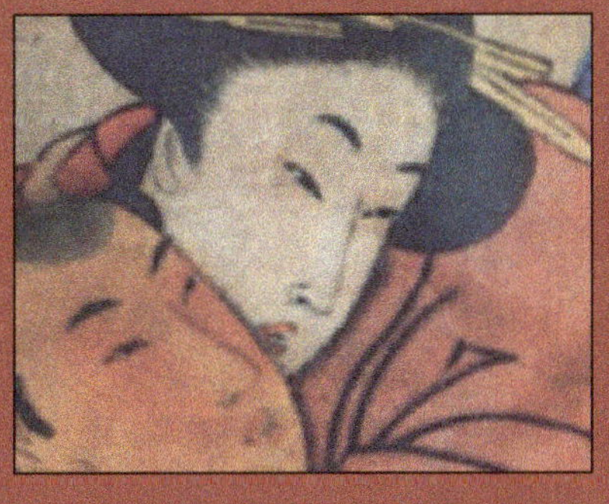

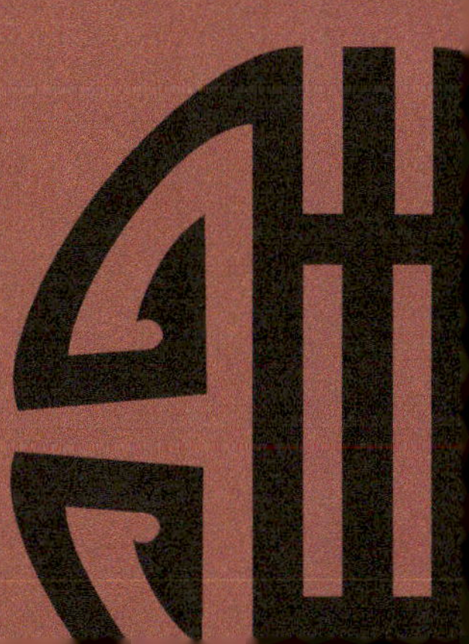

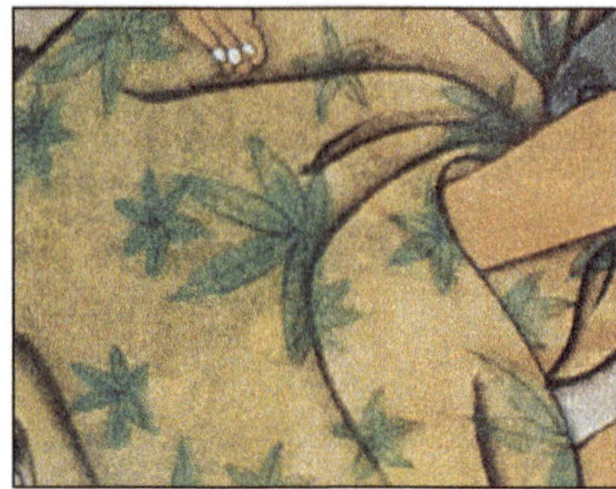

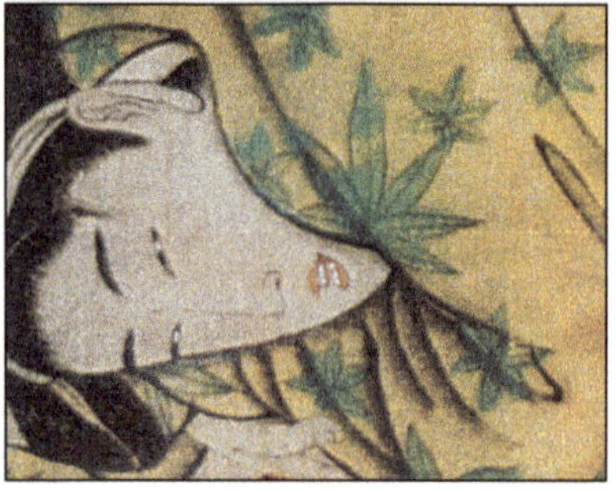

60

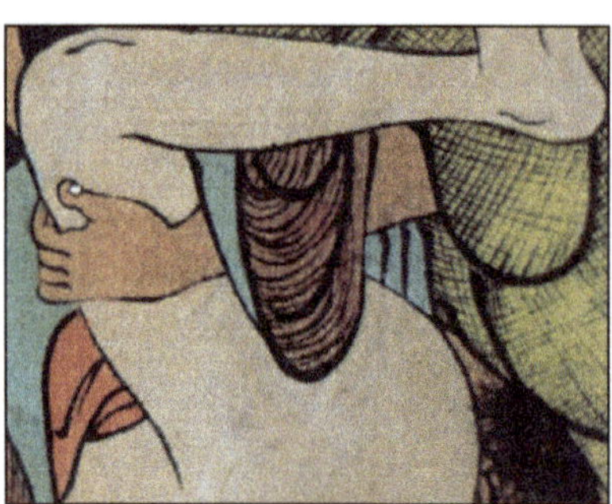

Utamaro (1753-1806), the absolute master of coloured woodcuts, divided his life between his art and the Yoshiwara district. Goncourt, who wrote his biography, wrote of him that 'He spent his days with his editor or in his studio and his nights in Yoshiwara.' Since his publisher's office was situated right at the entrance to the infamous district, the path between his studio and the houses of pleasure was doubtless a short one. Perhaps we could consider him a Japanese Toulouse-Lautrec?

There were 50 houses of ill-repute listed at that time, with nearly 6,000 girls, of whom at least 2,500 were courtesans offering various pleasures. Edo, which is now the city of Tokyo, numbered at the time over a million inhabitants. The greatest courtesans of the period owed the brilliance of their existence not only to the wealthy city bourgeoisie but also and especially to the large number of provincial aristocrats who had ended up in the capital. These were men with no occupation and nothing to do, and the hours they spent enjoying the pleasures of the Yoshiwara district made it easy for the police to keep them constantly under surveillance.

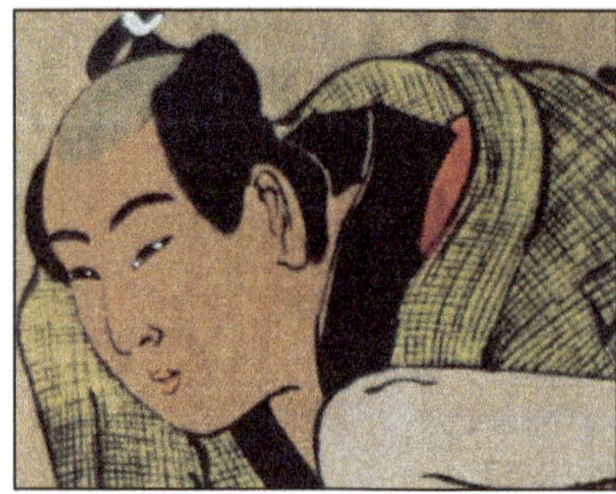

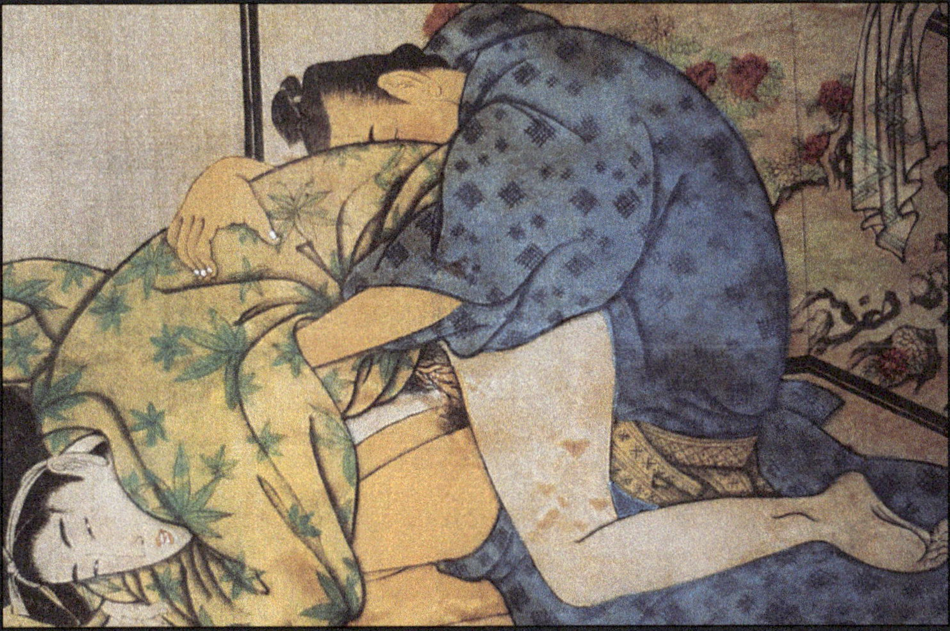

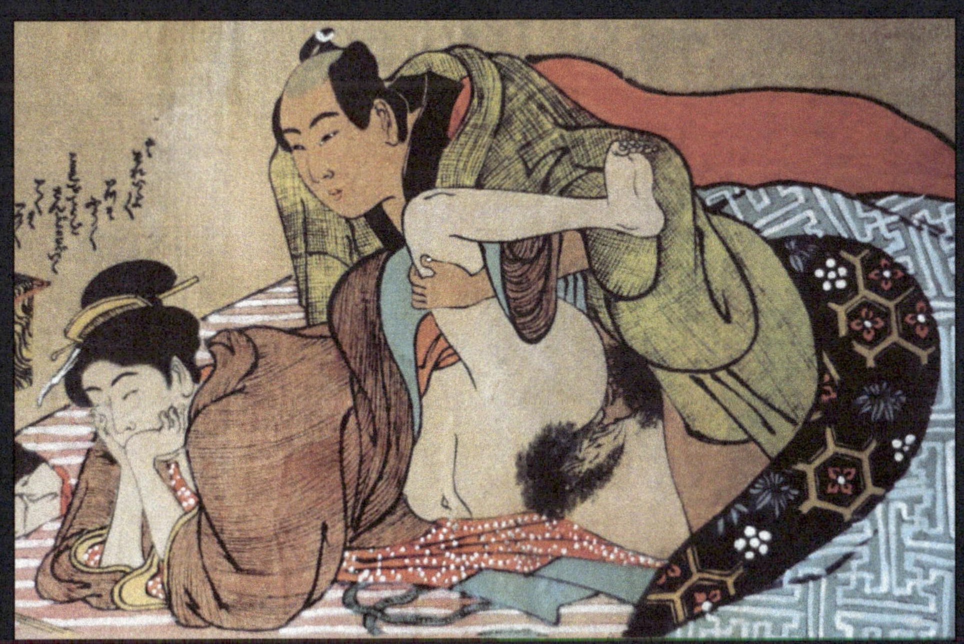

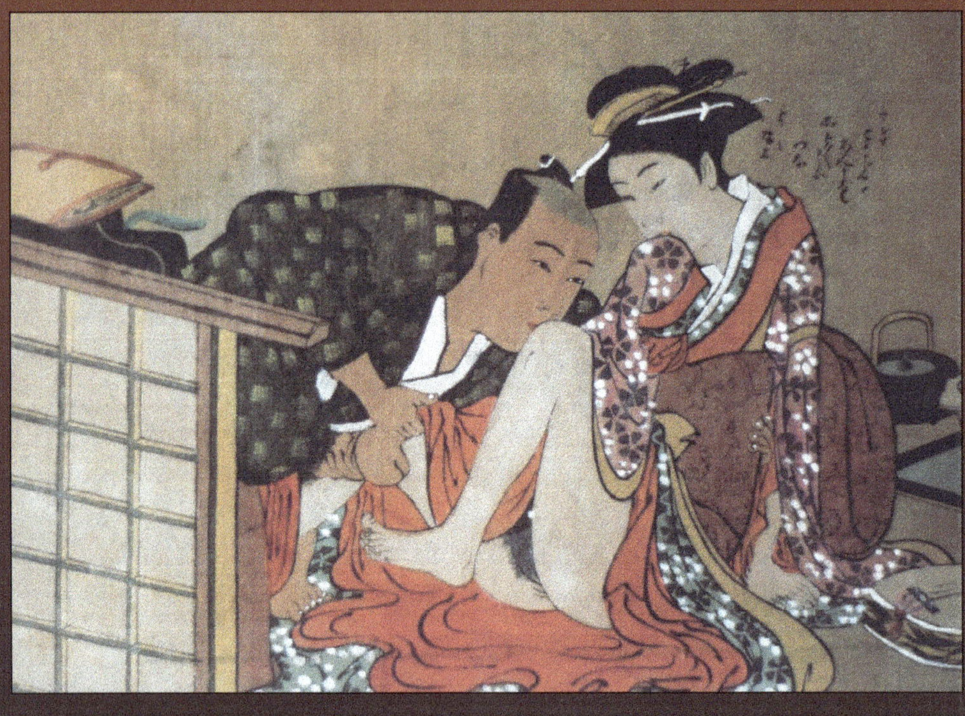

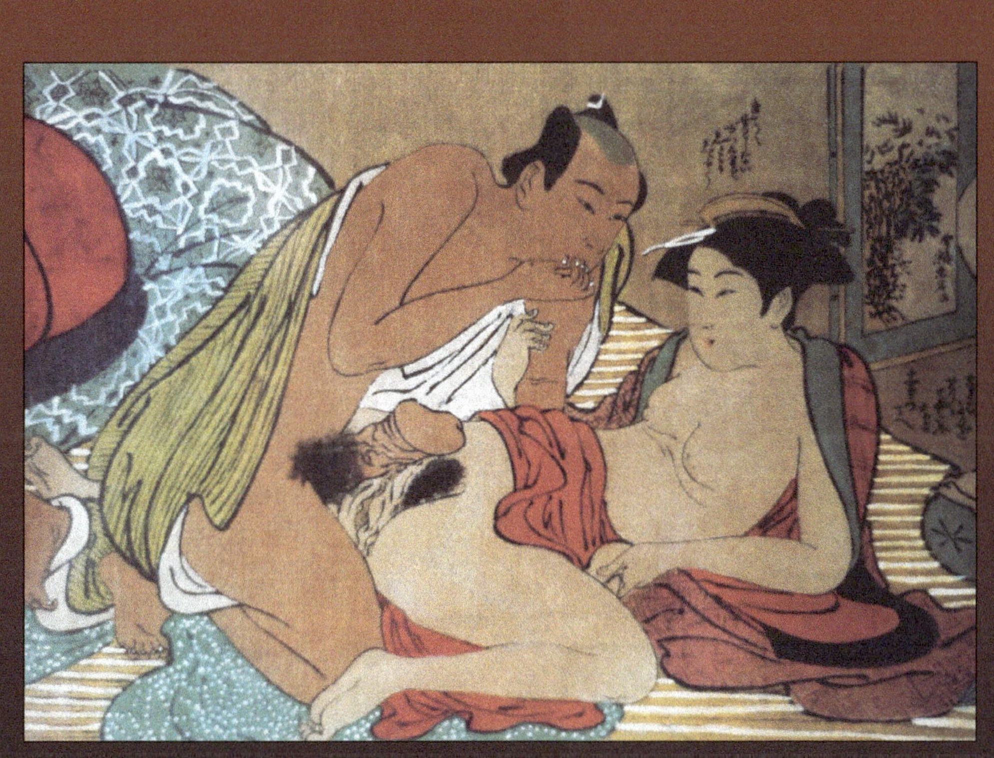

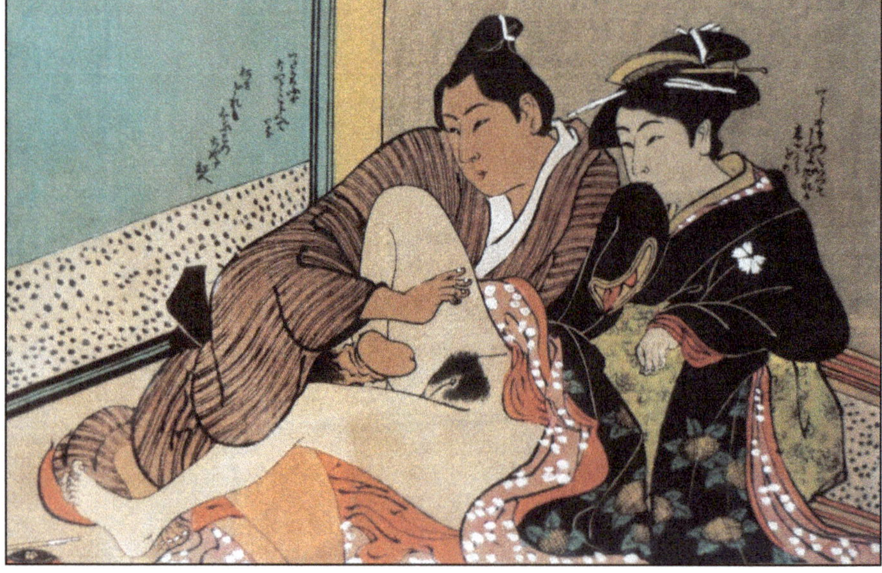

64

Just as European absolutism had declined in influence, so Japanese warrior ideology had lost an important part of its influence in Japan. Thus love and sexuality came to replace the more bellicose activities of the nobility. So when the noblemen moved around the capital with their numerous suites, they travelled regularly by horse to the Yoshiwara district or were carried there by litter. The state police had therefore not hesitated in granting a licence to the pleasure district; it made their task of surveillance much easier to have this group of individuals all in one place.

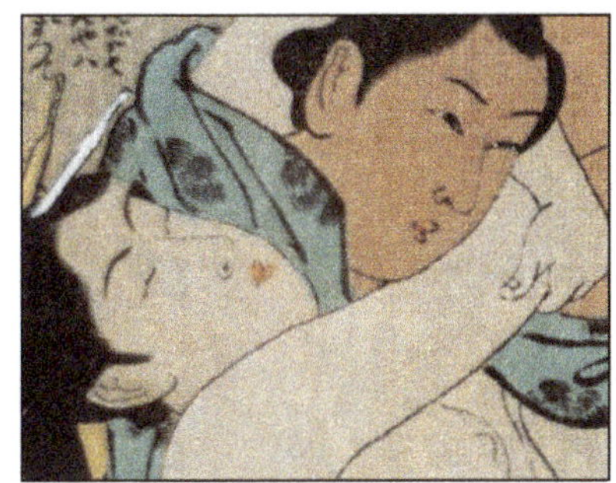

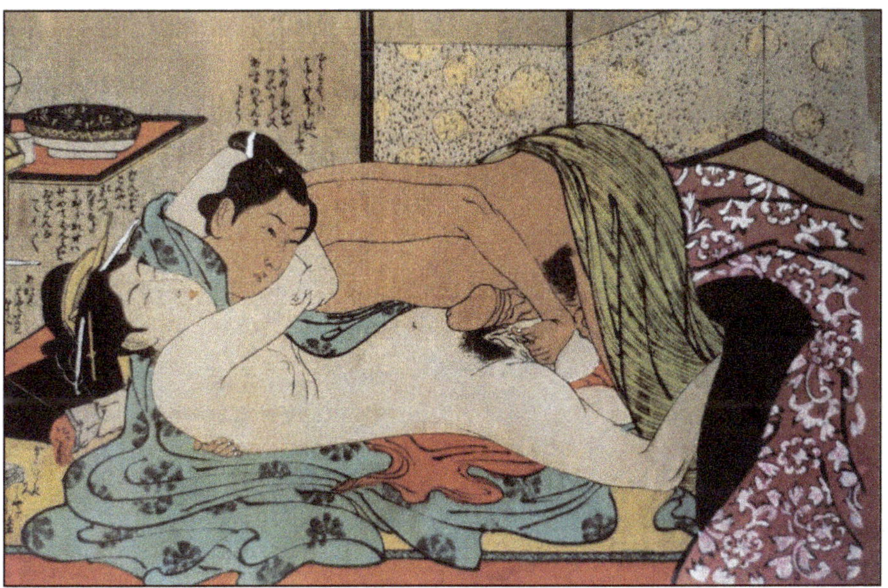

Yoshiwara was founded in around 1600 on marshy land – then known as 'rush land' – and was situated behind the imperial palace. In 1657, after the great city fire, it had to move to the area near the Merciful Temple of Asakusa, but its name remained unchanged. The district was then surrounded by walls and ditches and divided into nine separate areas. Entering this 'town of perpetual daylight which glitters resplendent like a peacock's tail', the first thing one would have encountered was the main street with its 50 tea houses which really did serve tea and nothing more.

65

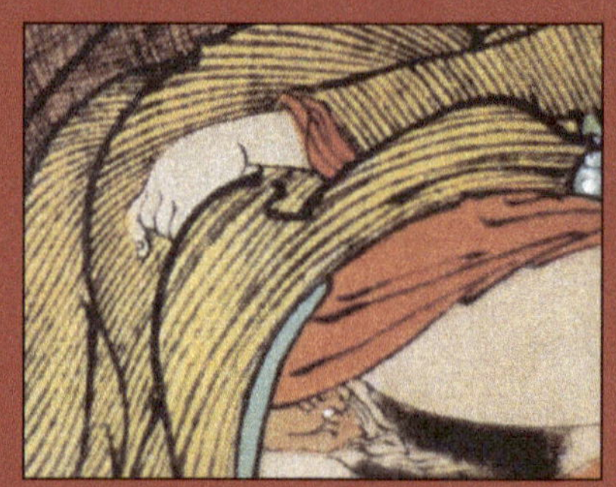

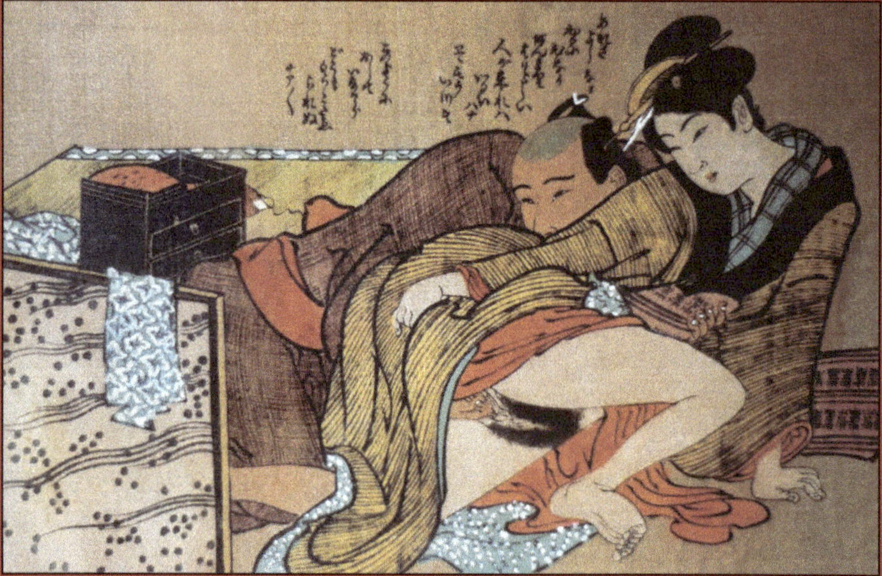

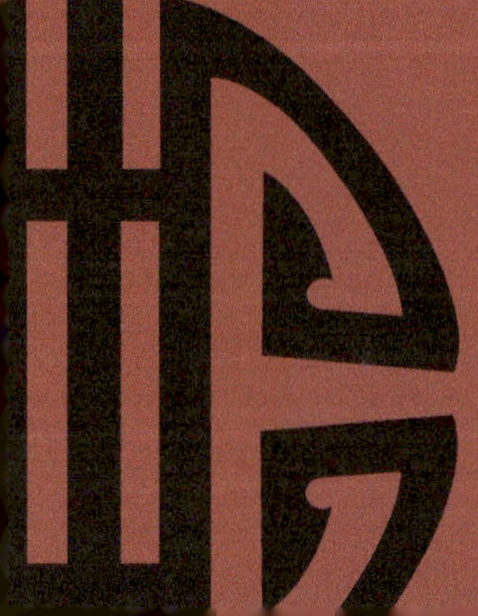

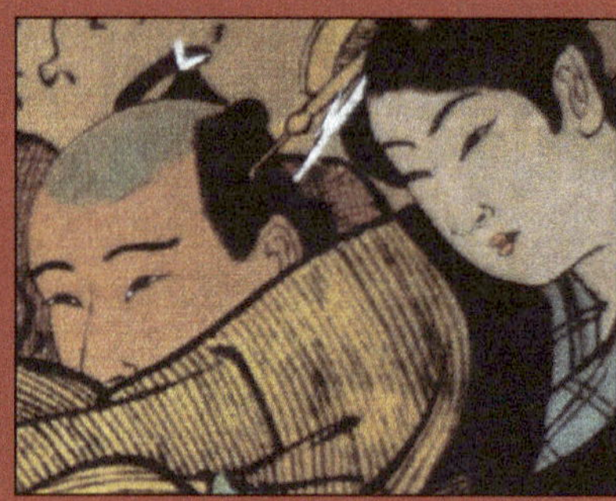

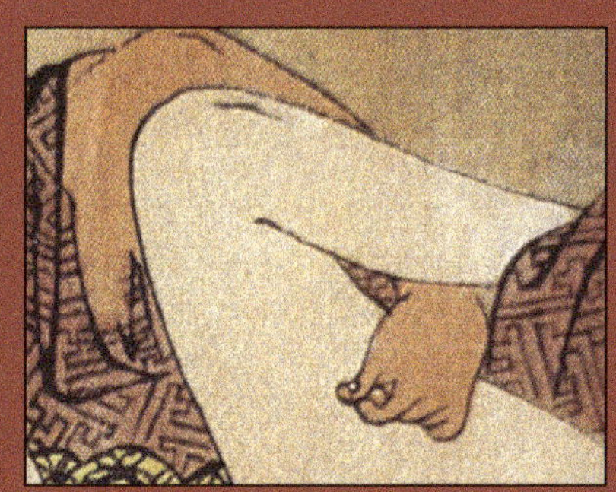

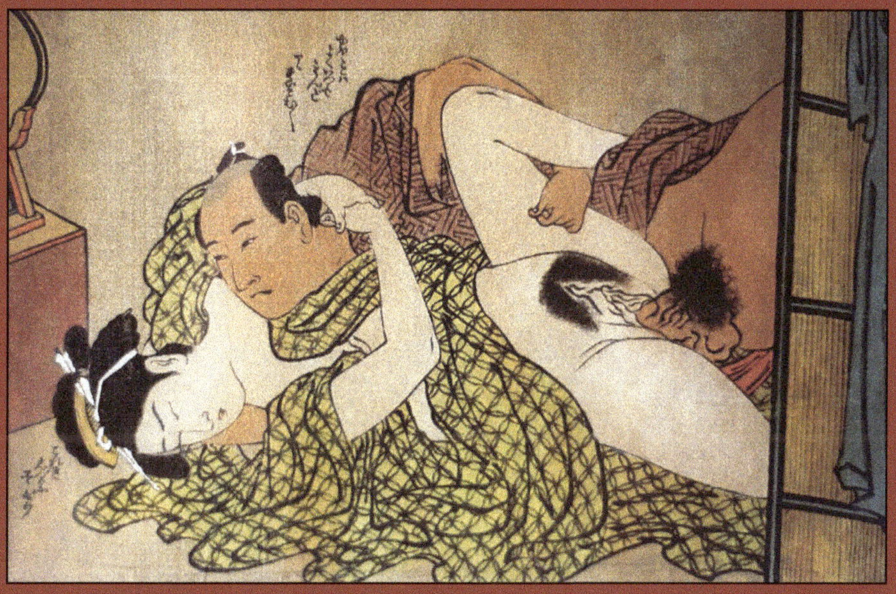

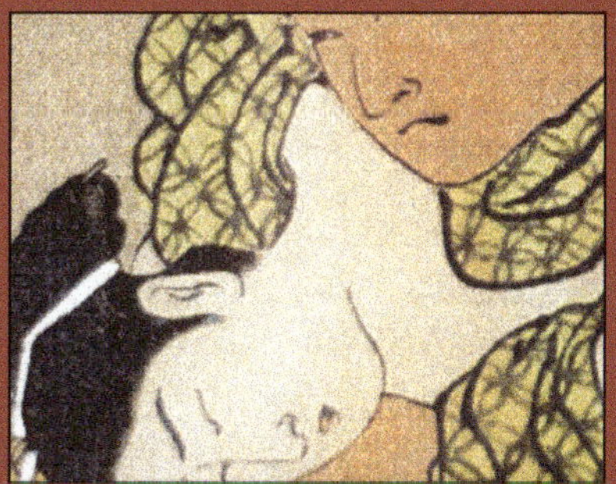

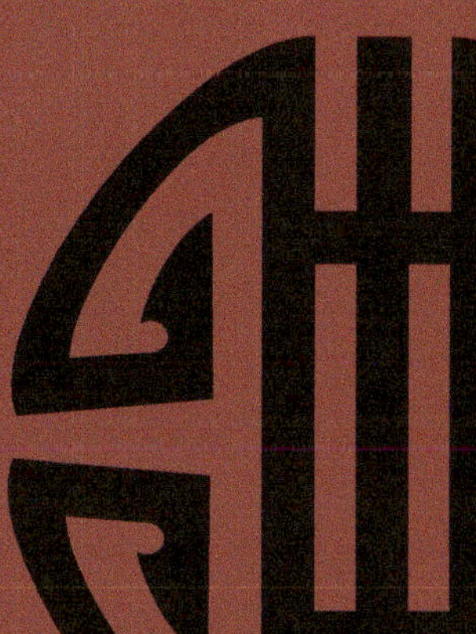

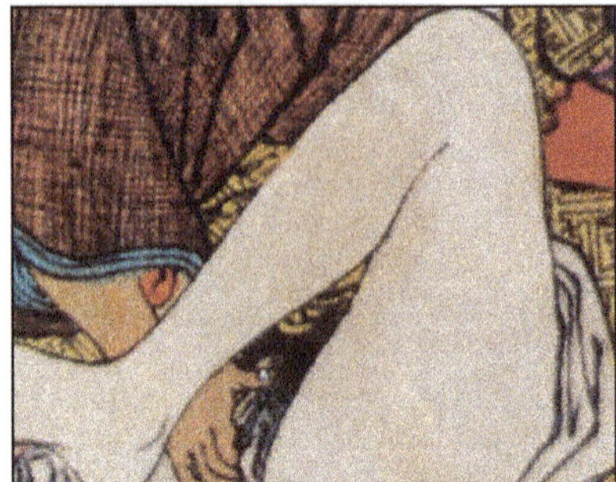

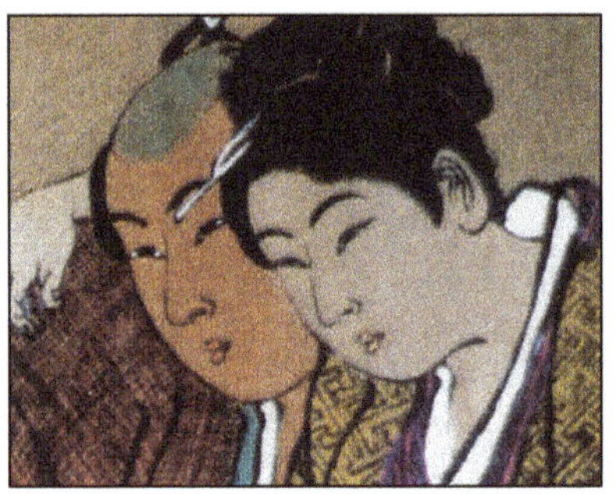

68

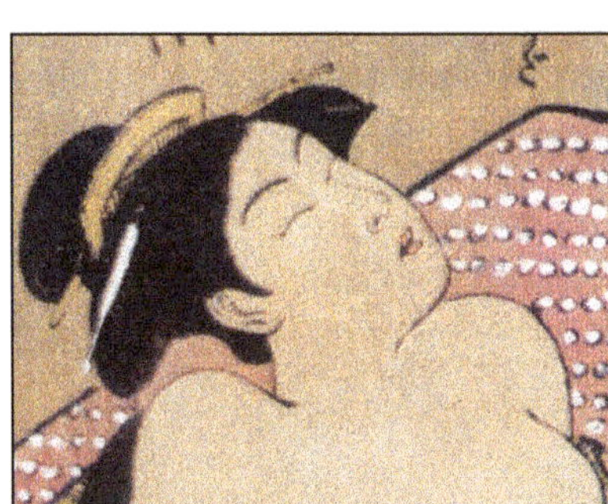

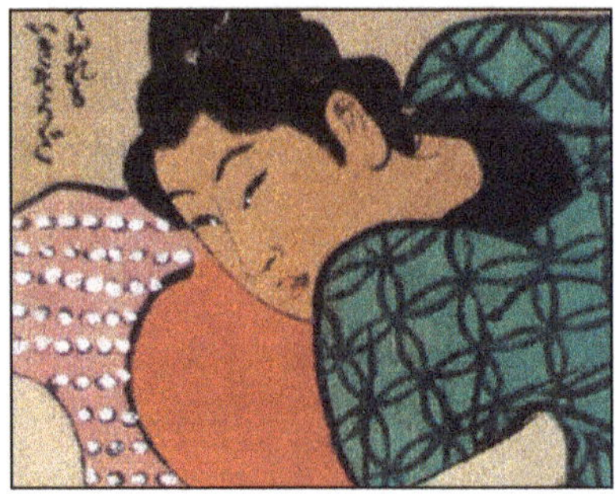

In a way, they acted as the antechambers to the brothels and as places where clients and prostitutes could meet and agree terms. Parties took place there and everything was so incredible and splendid 'one began to doubt whether one was still on earth.'

The 'library' of these 'houses of ill-repute' usually consisted of erotic books. As clients waited their turn, they would pass the time drinking tea and flicking through these albums with their risqué pictures and amusing stories.

As with the Greeks, so also for the Japanese physical love signified an elevated state of being. Like the Greek hetaera, the courtesans of Yoshiwara were proficient in different arts. They wore beautiful and costly garments, just like real princesses. Jippensha Ikku, a friend of Utamaro, once said of the women of Yoshiwara: 'They are educated like princesses. From a very early age they are given a full education. They know how to read and write, they learn all the arts, music as well as the tea ceremony, ikebana or the best way to arrange a bunch of incense.' At the beginning, the courtesans used to use an old-fashioned poetic language, as had been the custom in the imperial palaces over a thousand years earlier, but which no longer bore any resemblance to everyday Japanese.

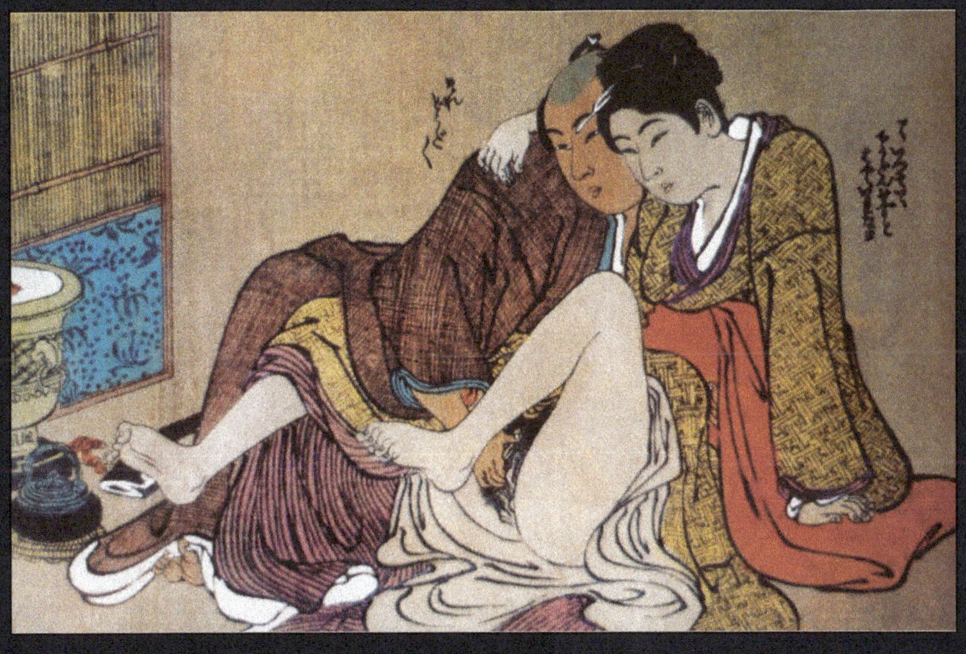
れんぼく
てうらしと
うらしらと
そのつる

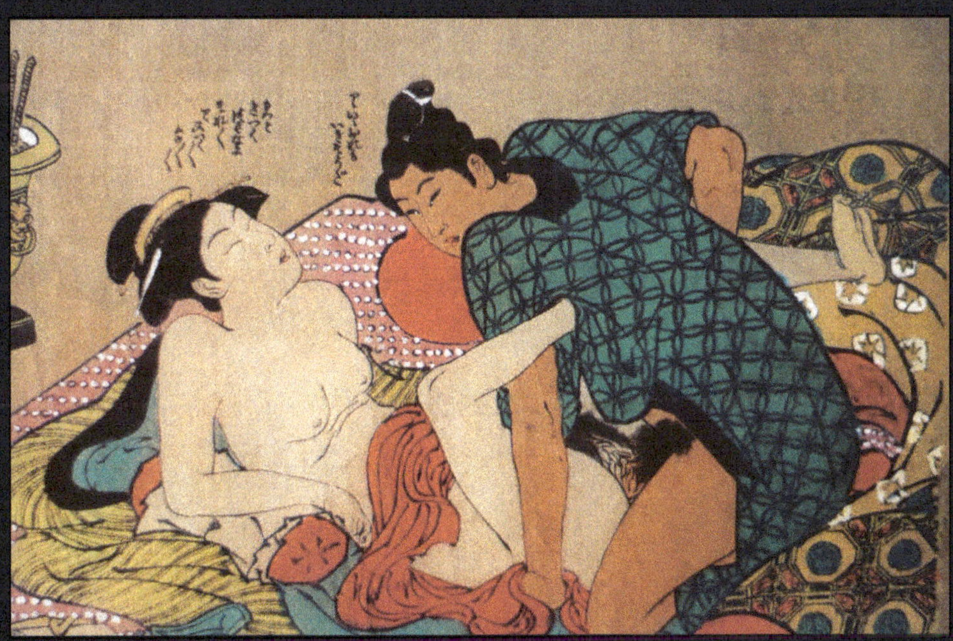
あれ
きやく
はいや
あら
あやく
てうら
うく
てうちをの
うらしやく

Japanese erotic engravings

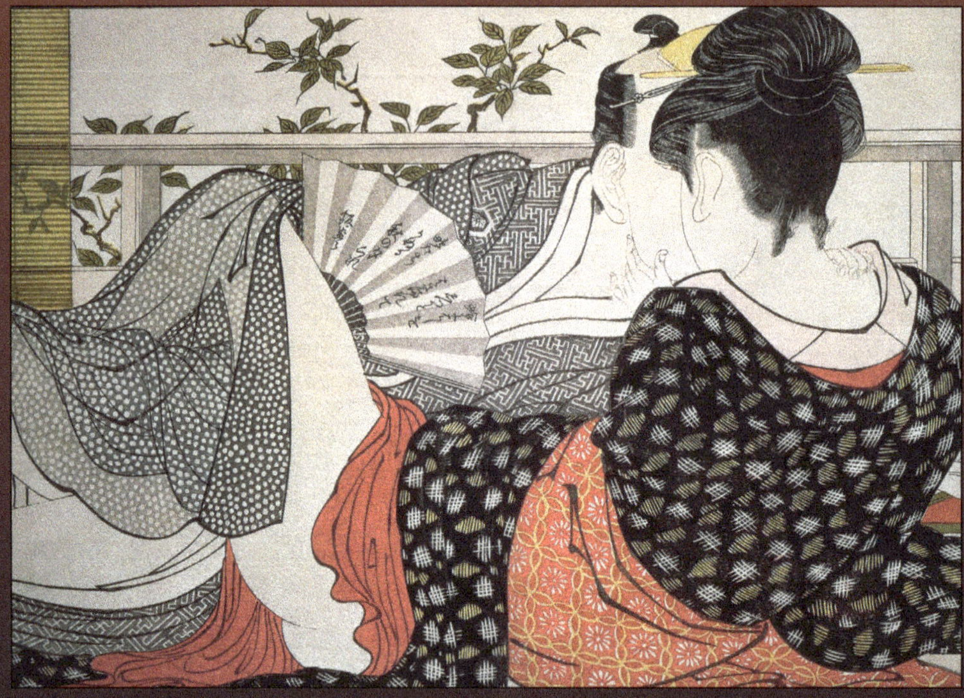

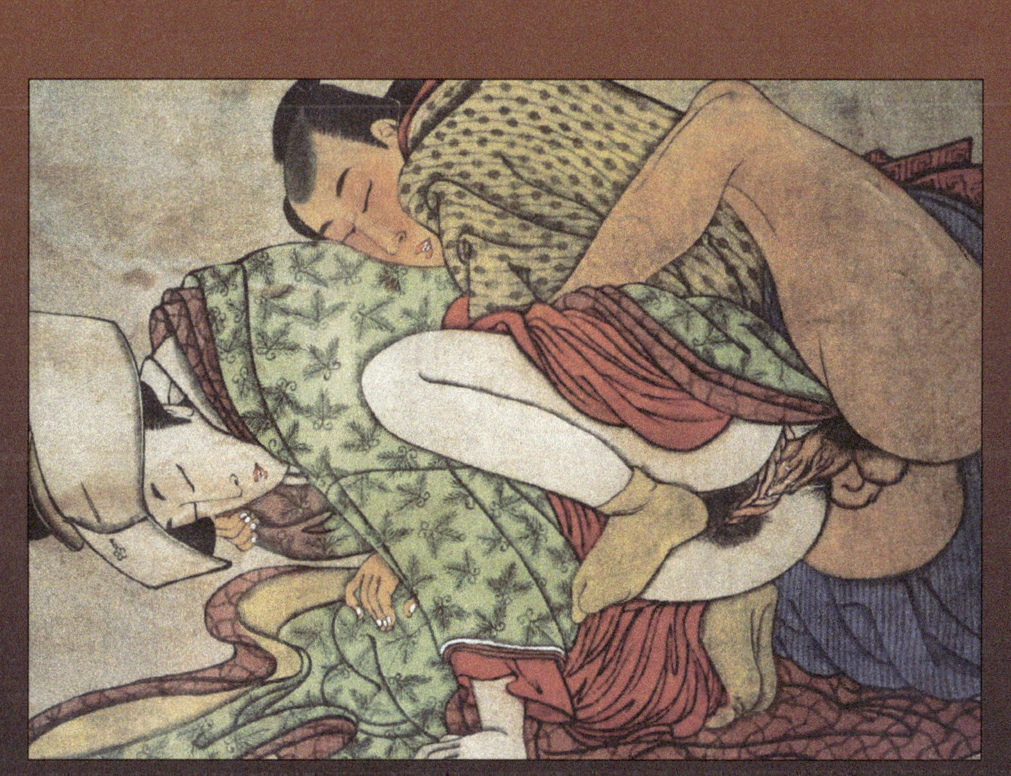

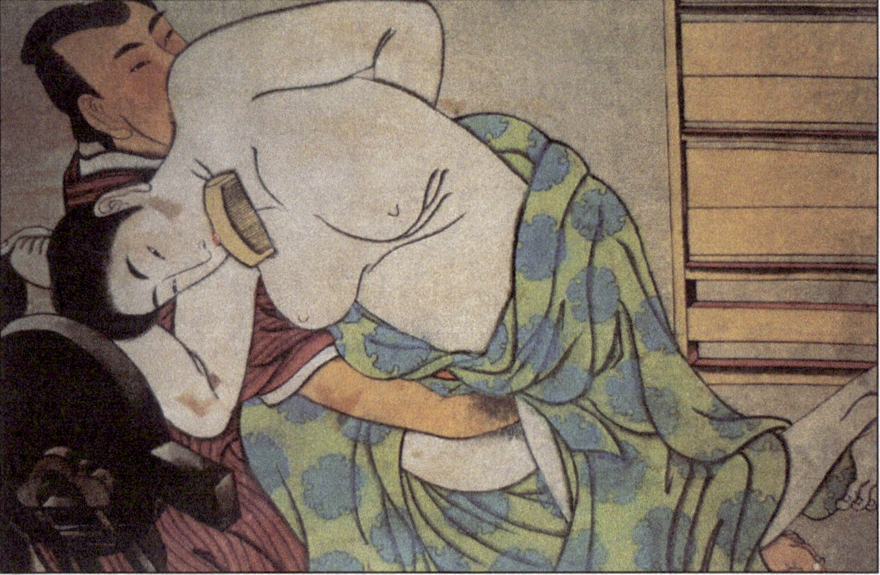

72

So, is the geisha a robot-like creature created solely for man's satisfaction? She is, as Théo Lesoual'h has remarked, the product of a long transformation wrought by the Japanese to the image of woman: the flawless form in which all elements of 'femininity' can be found condensed. Nothing in a geisha's behaviour is left to chance. In the eyes of the man, she is the symbol of perfection, from her refined and artistic hairstyle or her way of wearing make-up and wooden-soled sandals, right down to the perfectly-judged manner of her behaviour, which clearly dictated

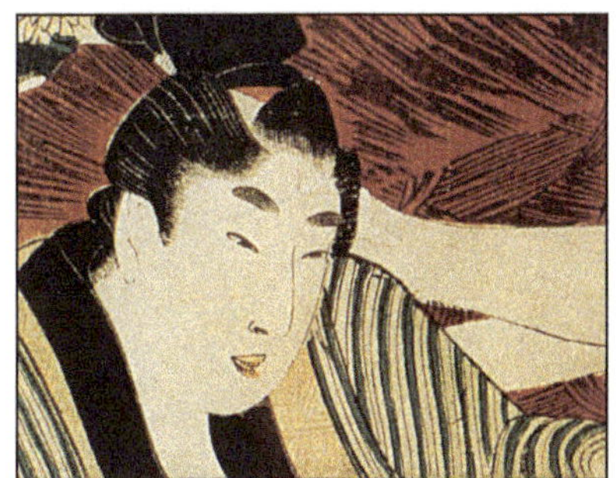

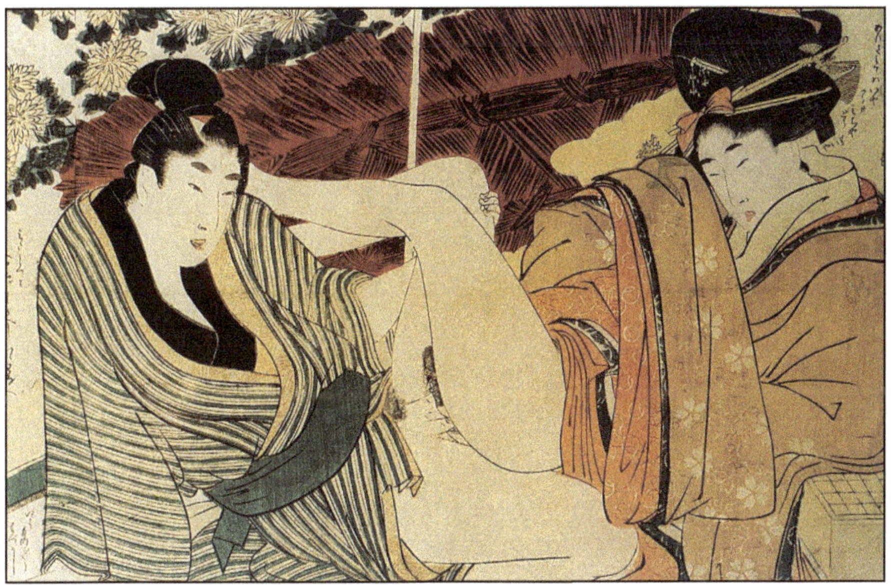

how she should position her body,
what her conversation should be
and how she should express her
feelings. 'The geisha is the
archetype of woman. She is the
erotic fetish of feminine grace,
although codified and reduced,'
wrote Lesoualc'h.

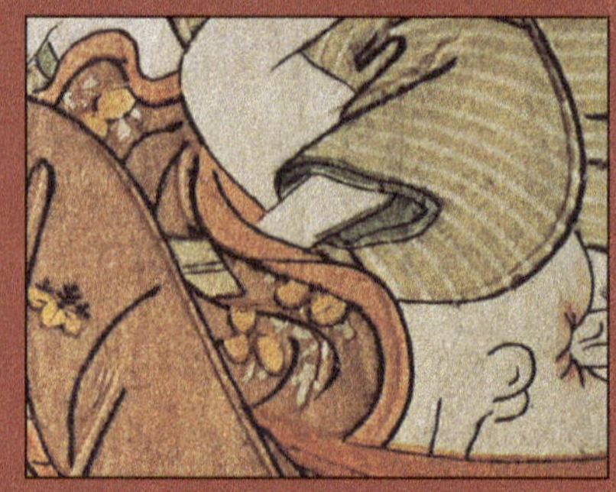

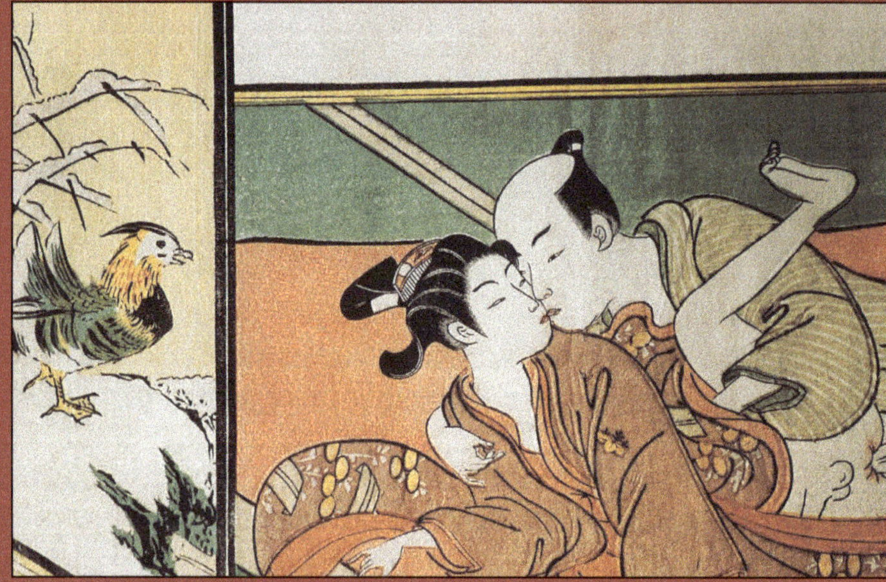

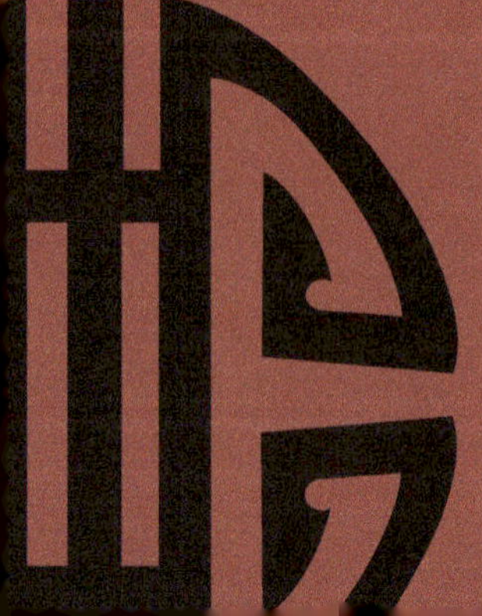

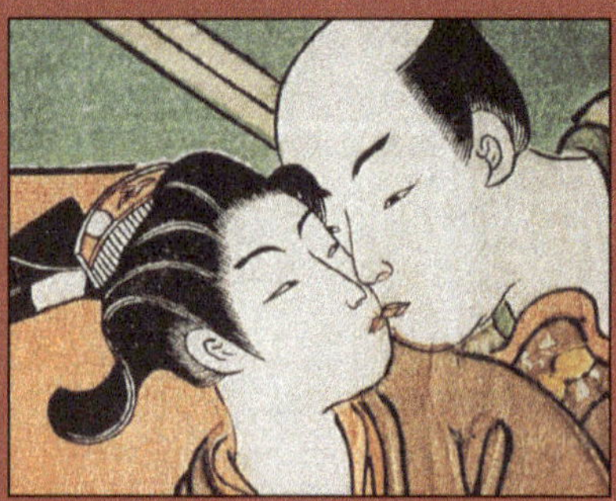

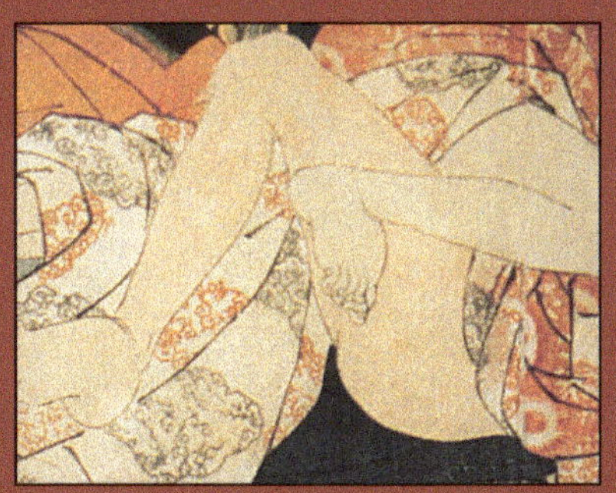

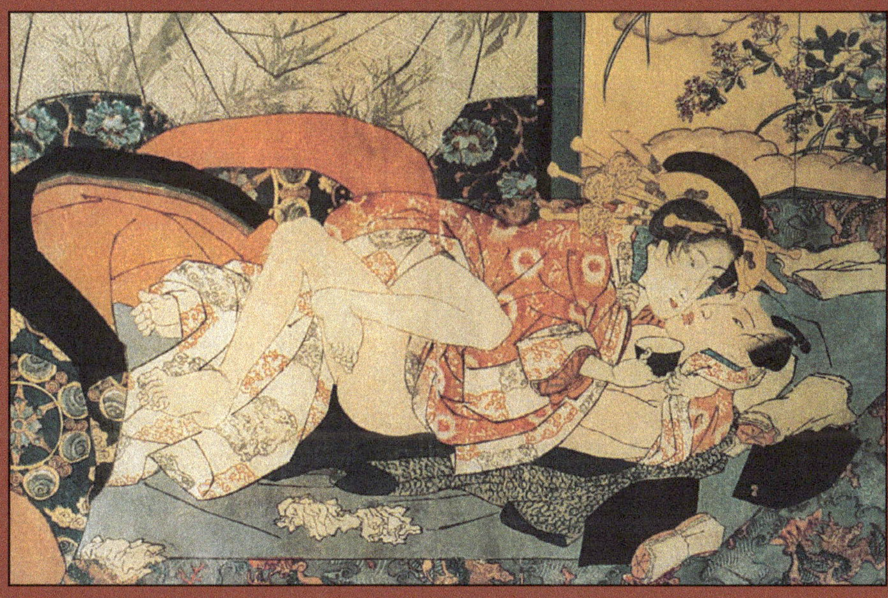

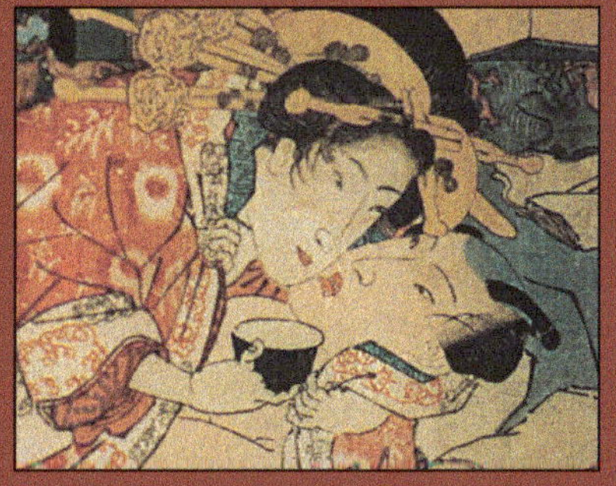

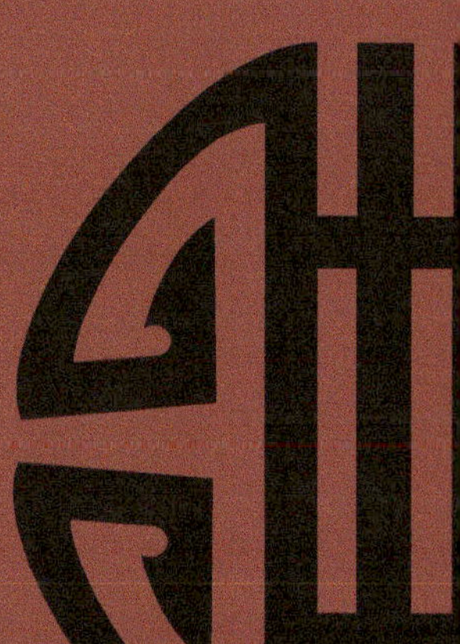

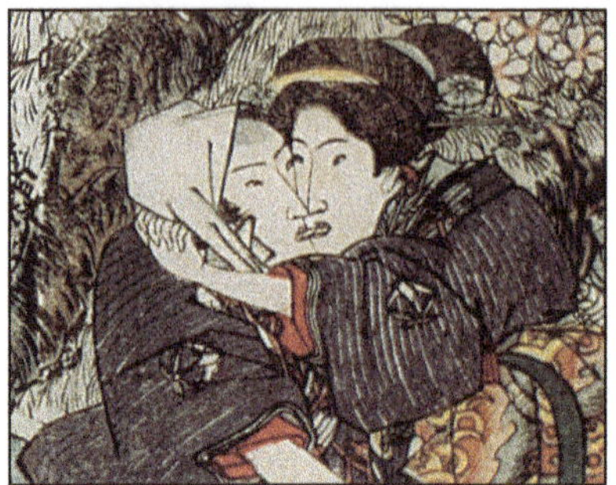

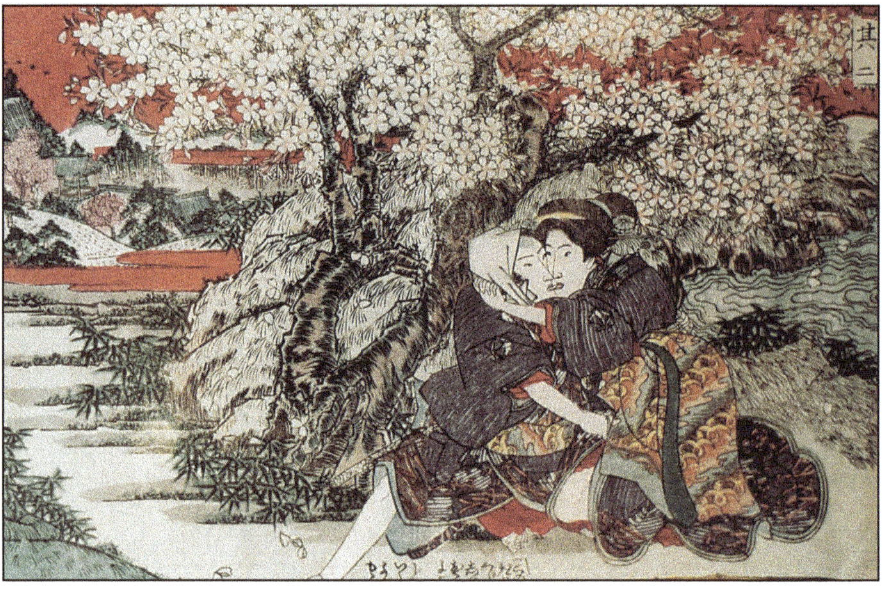

76

A Westerner looking at shungas will first of all notice the cold and detached expressions on the faces of the couples making love. Both sexes consummate the sexual act with a stoic impassivity, as if they were only partially involved in the act. Only their stretched-out and curled toes and the cloth which the woman bites with all her might to contain her excitement betray the extent of their ecstasy. Nothing which could possibly move the observer is expressed here, following the traditional rules of art.

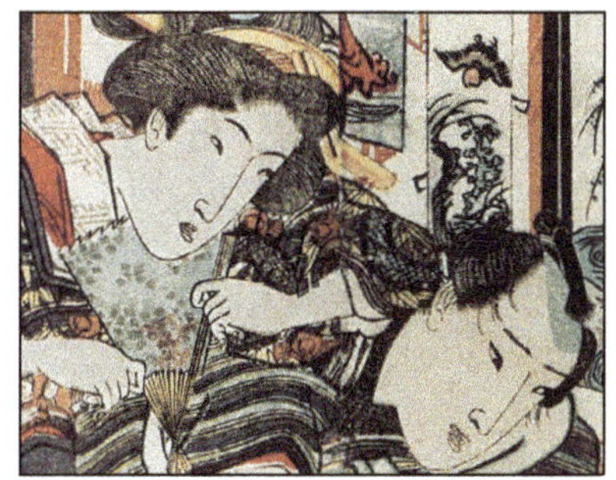

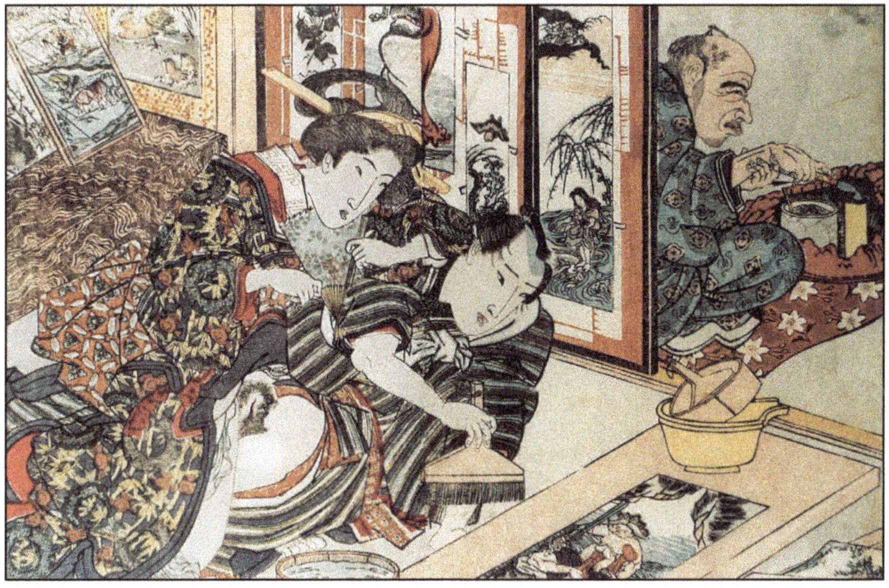

One might also notice the extremely exaggerated, almost caricature-like dimensions of the male organ. Could it be a fear of impotence that lies behind these over-inflated penises? Or is it the product of a fantasy which itself hides man's fear of woman's untamed nature? However, what we also find in these over-sized penises are reflections of the ancient phallic cult of the Shinto religion. Shintoism, which is the indigenous religion of Japan and a cult entirely devoid of all metaphysical dogmas, is an astonishing mixture of the most varied rituals in honour of over 800 polymorphic gods.

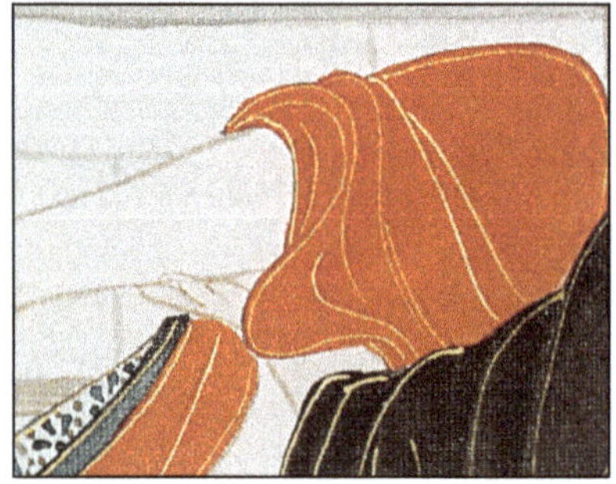

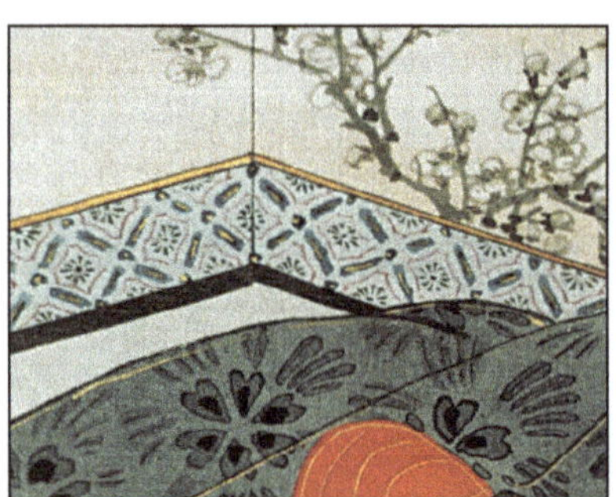

78

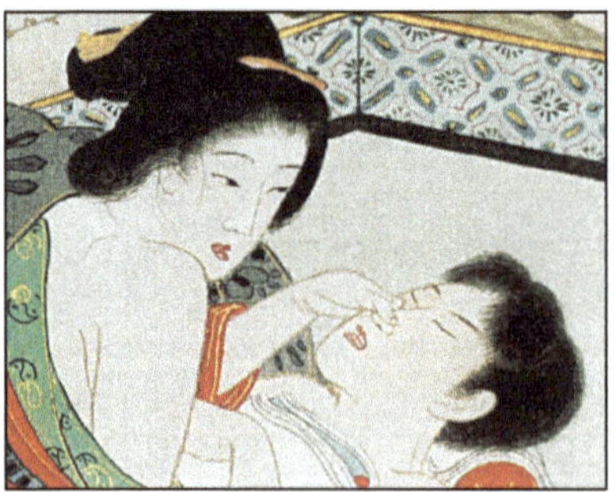

Thus the phallus quite naturally became a god to whom temples or private altars at home were dedicated. It was even invoked in prayer some evenings in the pleasure districts during the 17th and 18th centuries. Even today one can still come across ancient phallic steles on the edges of fields, placed there as a symbol of fertility. Festivals in honour of the phallus were a regular event and were the occasion for exuberant processions. An account dating from the end of the 19th century describes one of these processions in Tokyo: 'A phallus several metres high, all covered in gleaming varnish, was placed on a sort of portable casket and carried by a group of young men, who were shouting or laughing at the tops of their voices. They zig-zagged along the streets and made sudden, unexpected charges in all directions. Real bacchanalian rites!' Thus the cult of the phallus was the backbone of the Shinto religion. In the temples, wooden, porcelain, stone or metal phallic figures were sold as good-luck charms.

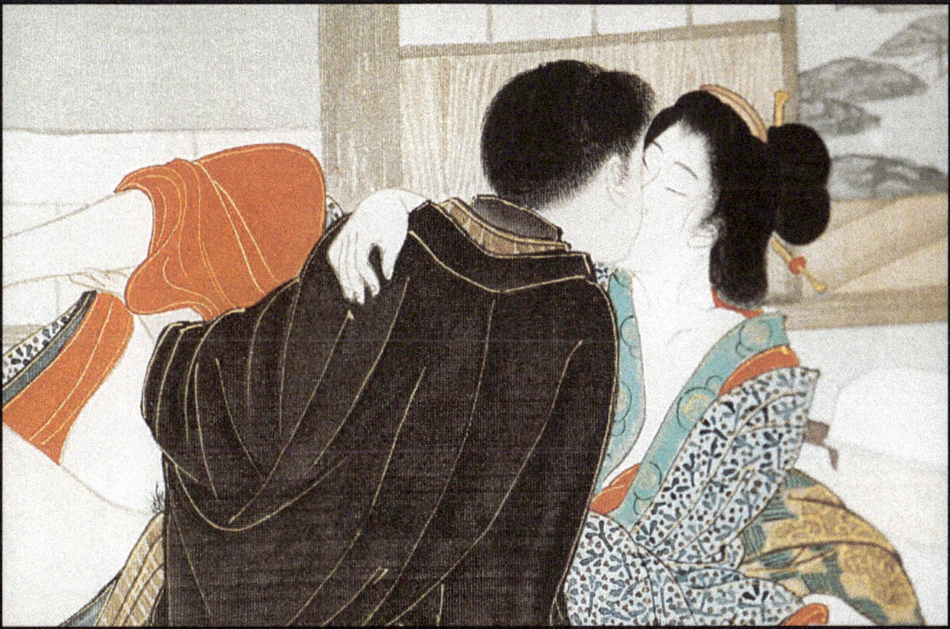

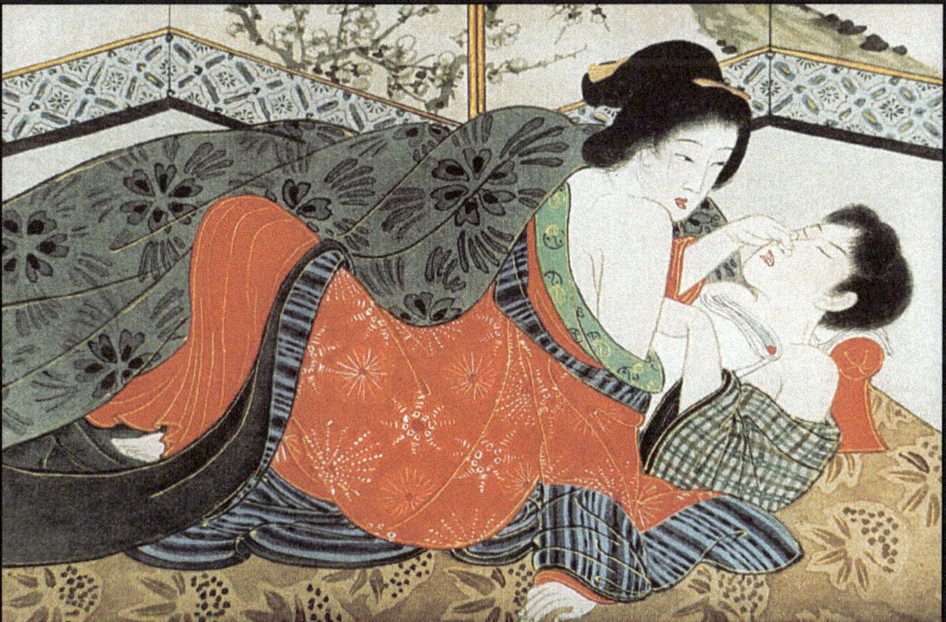

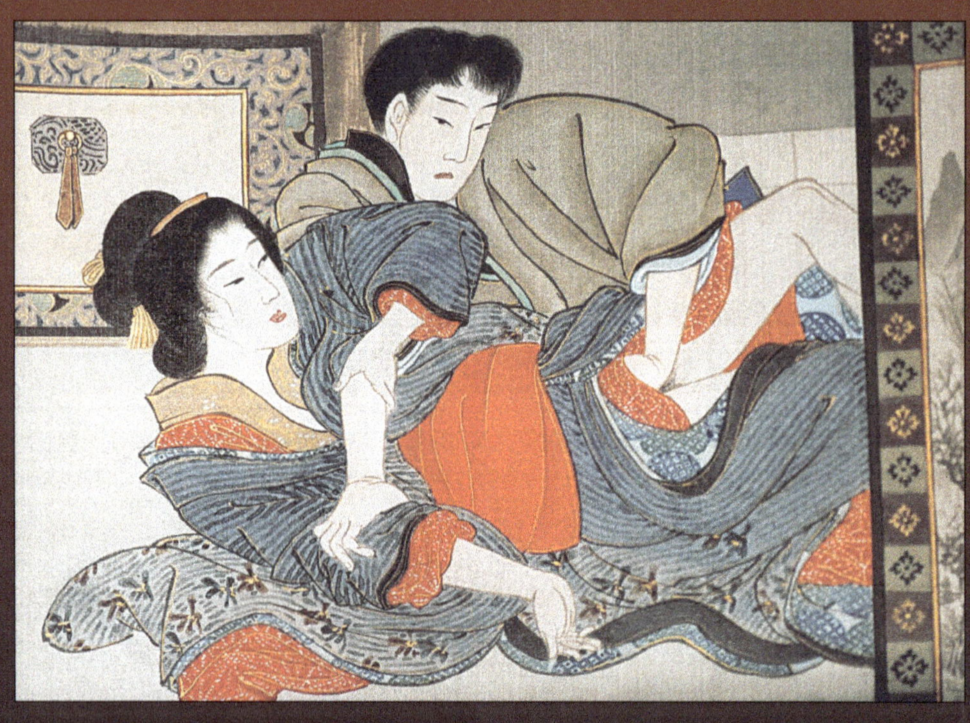

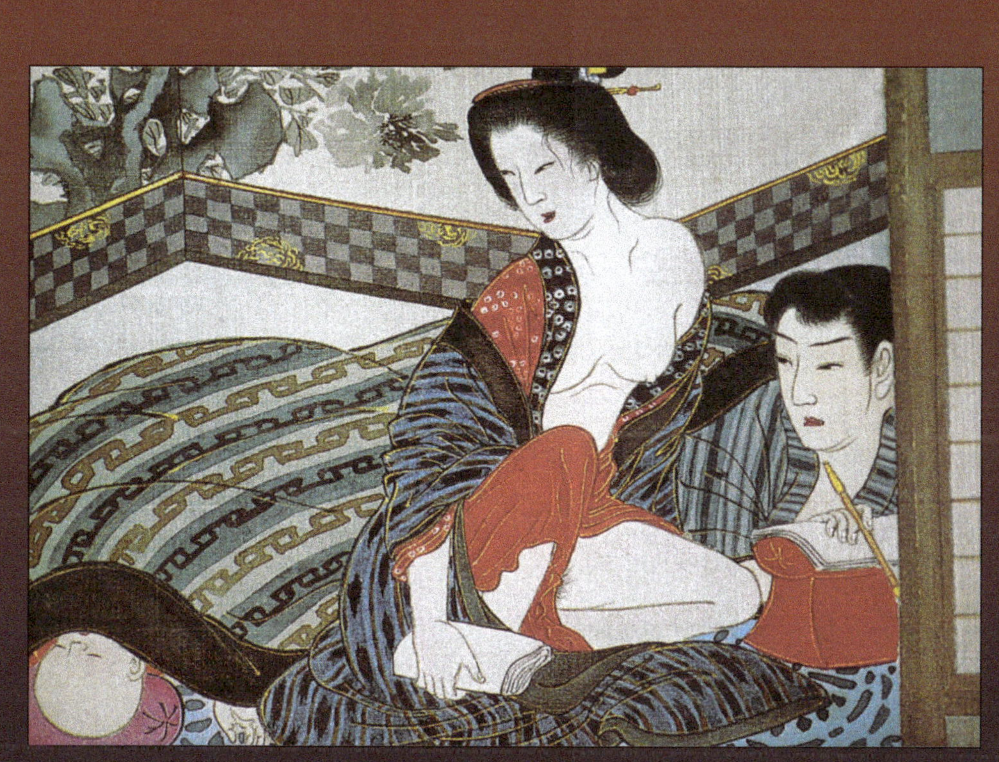

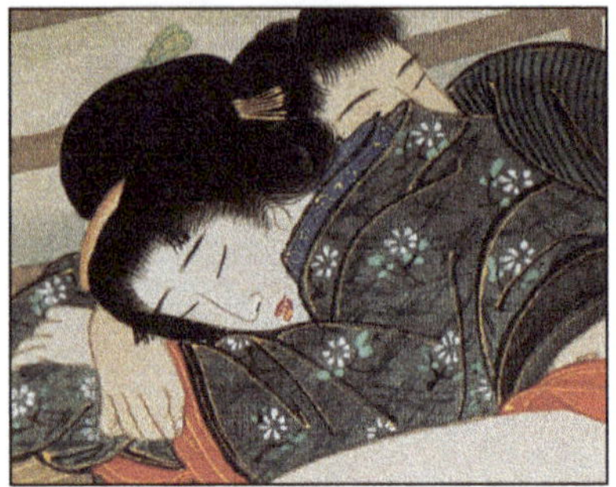

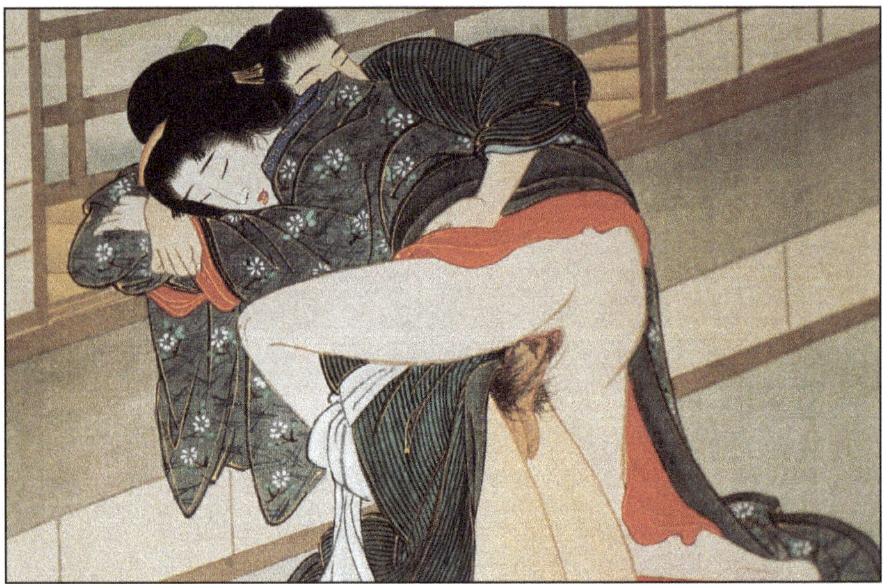

82

Japan never suppressed sensuality as such; if there were laws and limitations, they were always socially based but never religious. To seek physical pleasure was considered a natural desire, even if it consisted of unusual practices. Thus, sodomy figured among the normal pleasures of the body. The word 'sin', it seems, was never uttered. Even when we are shown 'natural love' in its many varied forms in the woodcarvings, they always involve massive priapic fantasies.

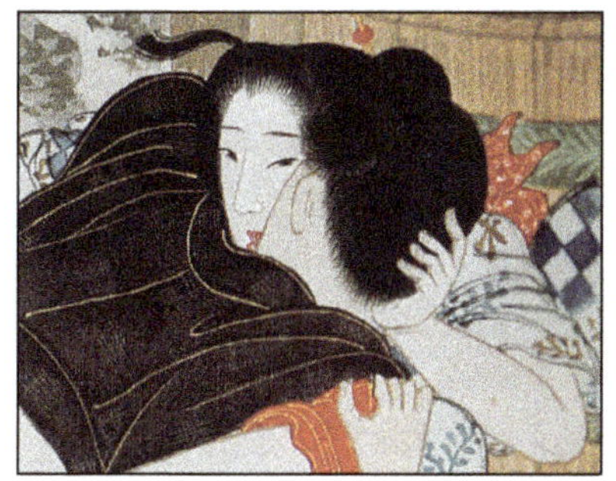

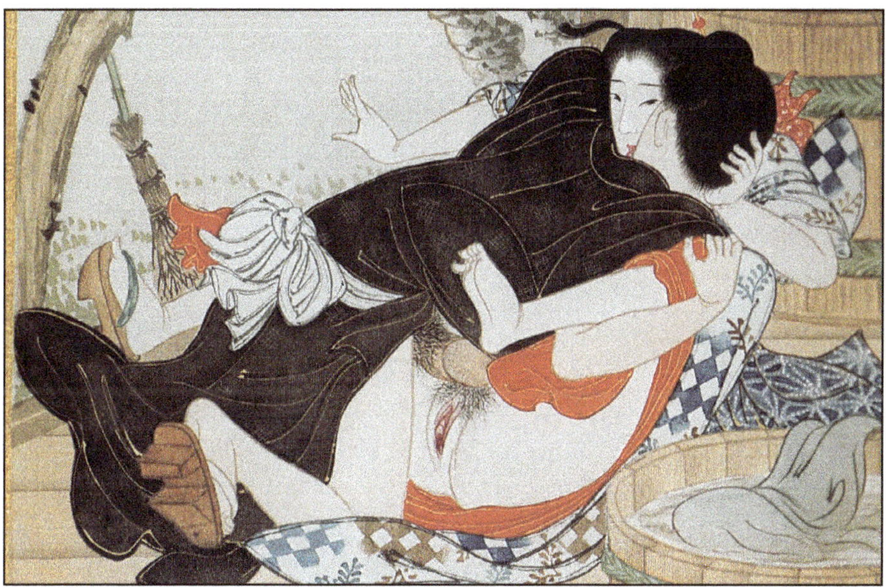

Almost all masters of woodcarving produced erotic images, sometimes even in such precious materials as gold, silver or mother-of-pearl. And yet the shunga studios were for the most part clandestine. Artists did not sign their work, or else used a pseudonym. The number of copies made was always limited and most often sold on the black market.

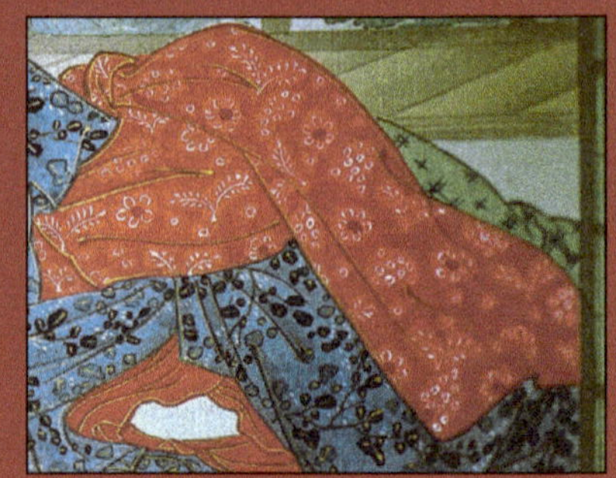

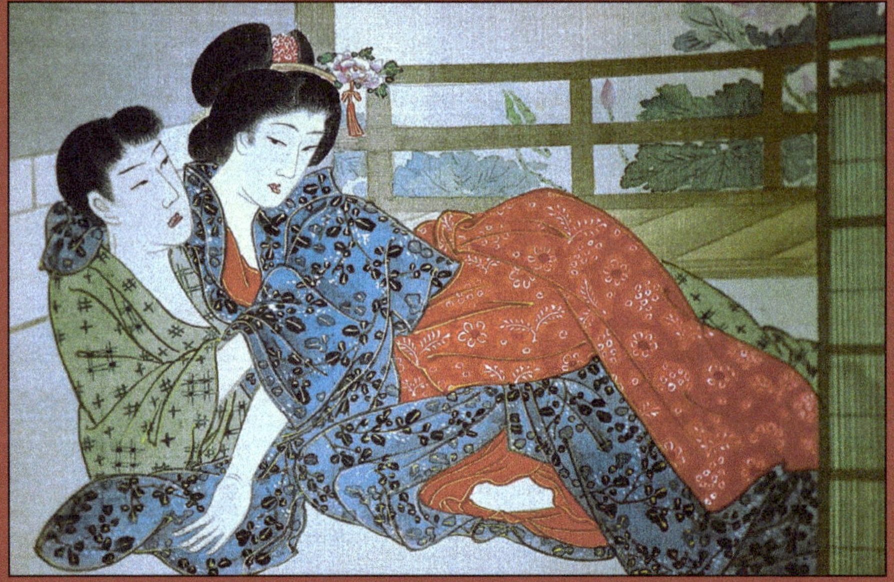

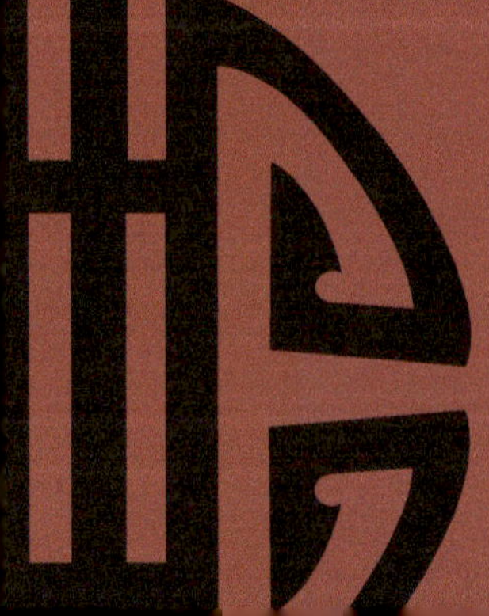

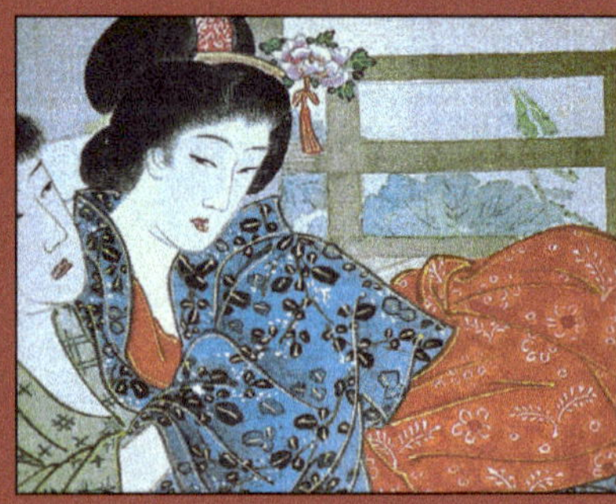

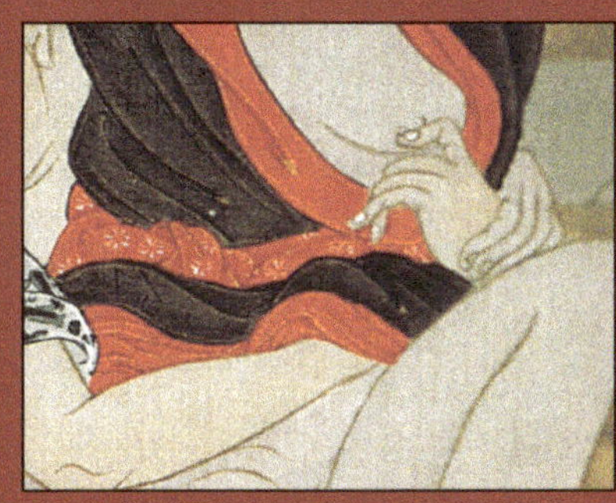

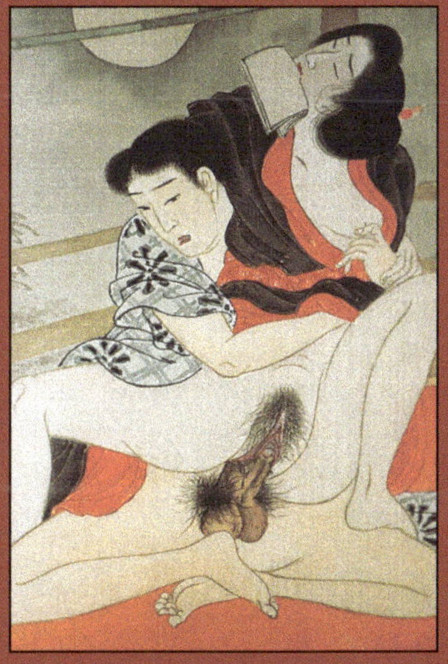

Purity of line became a rule that could not be broken for woodcarving; the artist had to carve out the lines in the wood with extreme care. Parallel perspective was mainly dominant: lines that were parallel in nature were also parallel in the wood. Central perspective, which was a European invention, was only introduced in the 19th century. Likewise, the Japanese were not familiar with the effects of shadow and light which are so much a part of European art. The initial technique was to print onto paper from one sole block and then to colour them by hand, which considerably restricted the numbers in which they could be produced because of the time involved. For this reason, in the 18th century, they started using several blocks.

Katsushika Hokusai (1760-1848) is the last great figure of the Ukiyo-e. After him, woodcarving began to decline, giving way to vulgar copies produced in large numbers and designed to cater to the tastes of the masses. By the second quarter of the 19th century, it had to all intents and purposes become a popular art.

85

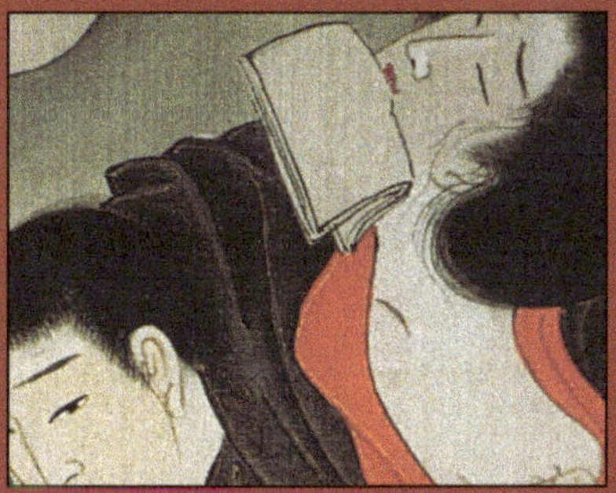

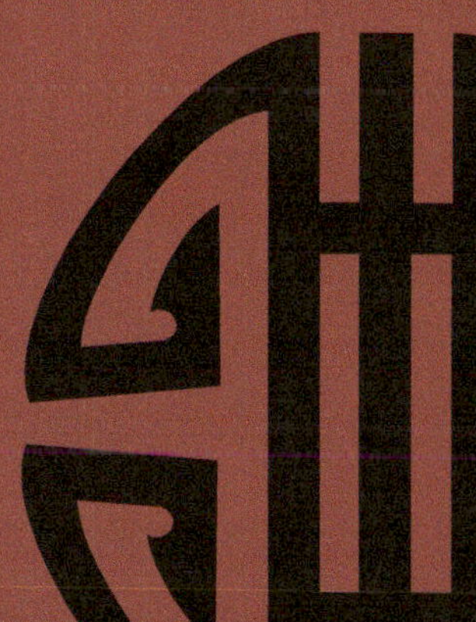

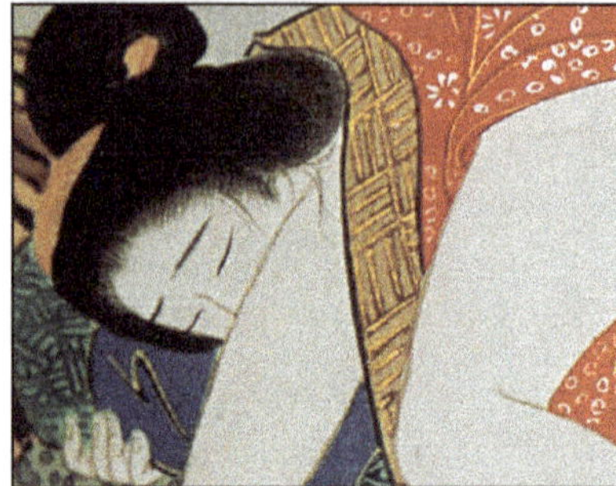

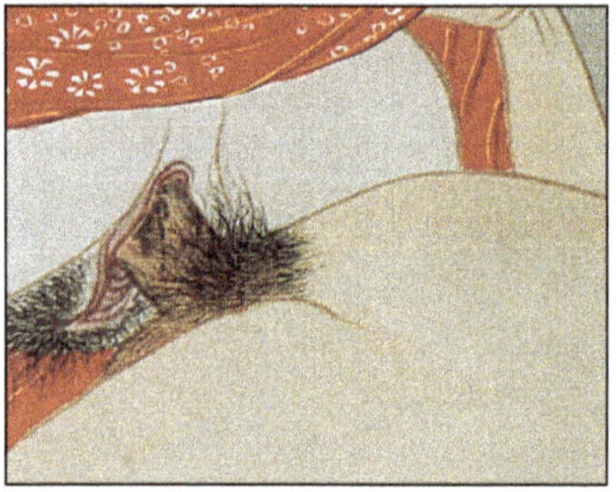

86

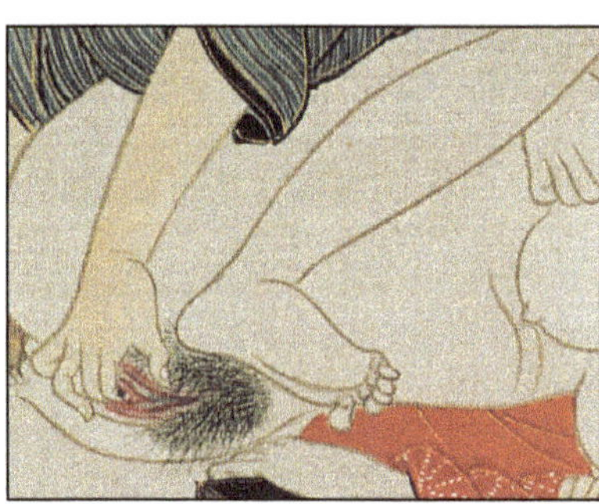

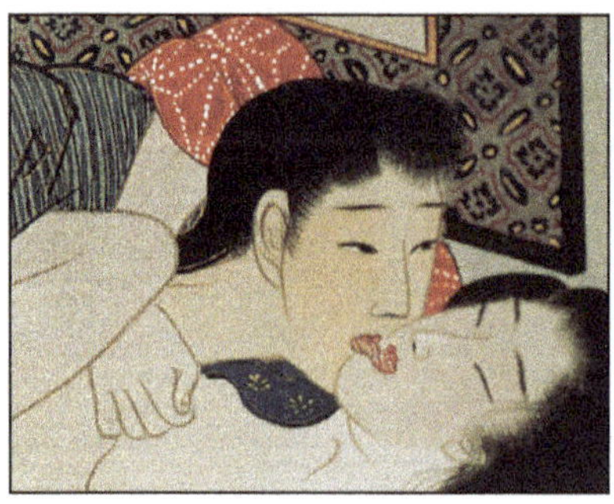

For a long time, Europe ignored Ukiyo-e on the grounds that its content went beyond the boundaries of good taste. It was not until the universal exhibitions in Paris of 1867, 1878 and 1889 that a western audience had the opportunity to rediscover an art form that had hitherto been despised. After that, none would dare deny the major influence of Japanese woodcarving on the entire Impressionist movement.

The English artist Aubrey Beardsley probably possessed the finest collection of Ukiyo-e and shunga. His work, which is so characteristic of the late 19th century, is a perfect illustration of the influence of Japanese woodcarving on western art.

Toulouse-Lautrec also possessed a remarkable collection, a few photographs of which remain. These prints, with their images of cruel and violent ghosts, seem to have particularly affected him, especially the scenes where women are embraced by animals, monkeys, foxes, badgers or vampires.

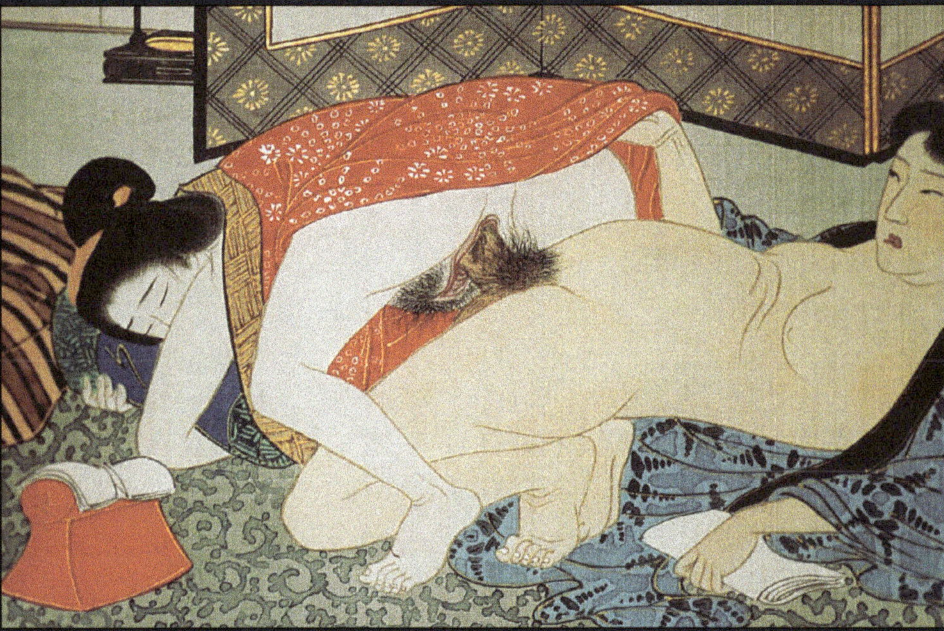

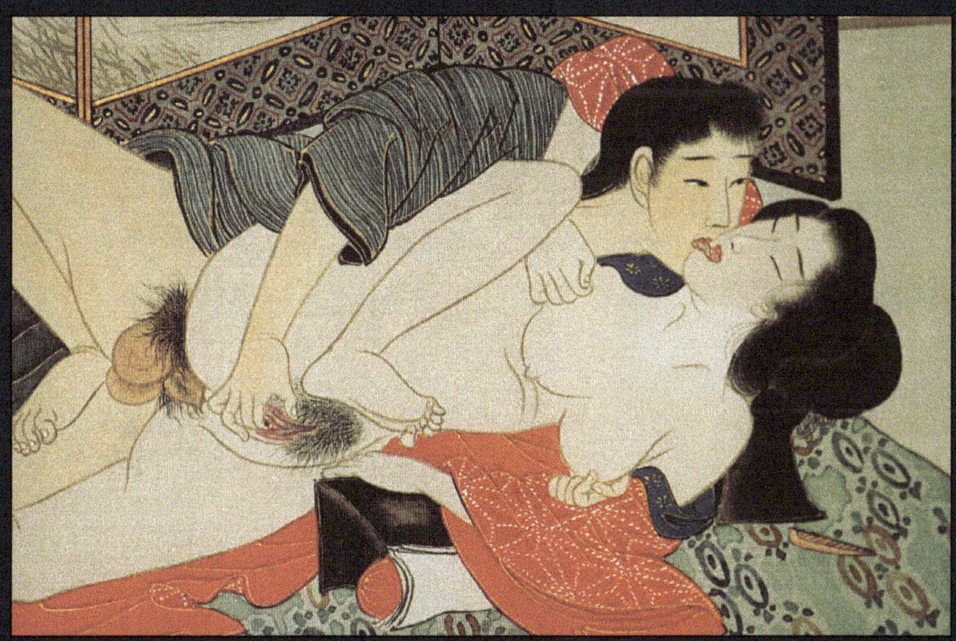

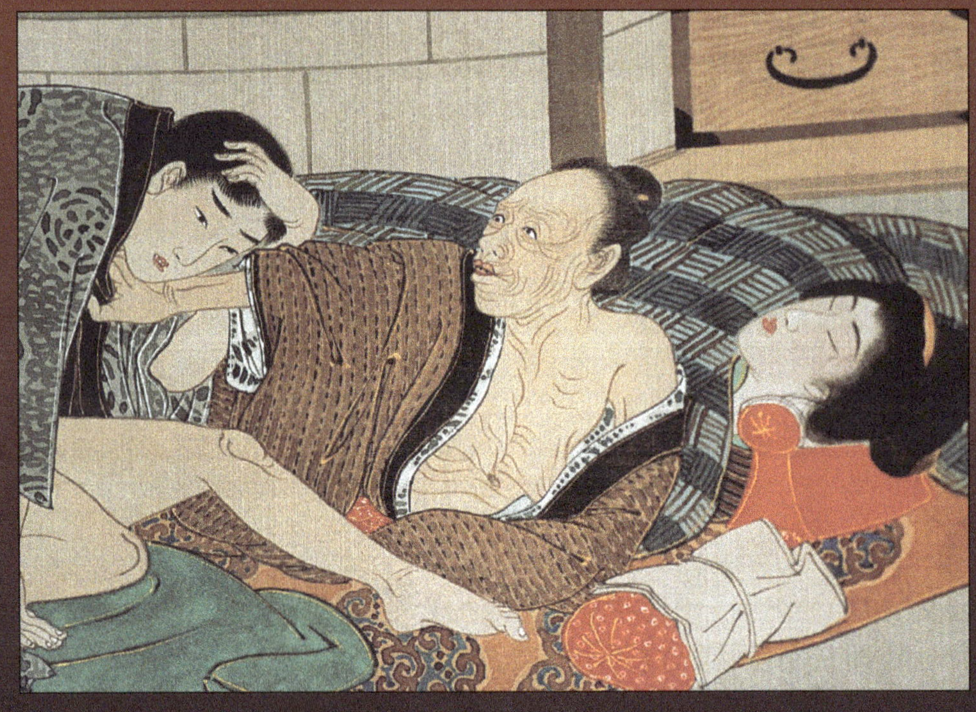

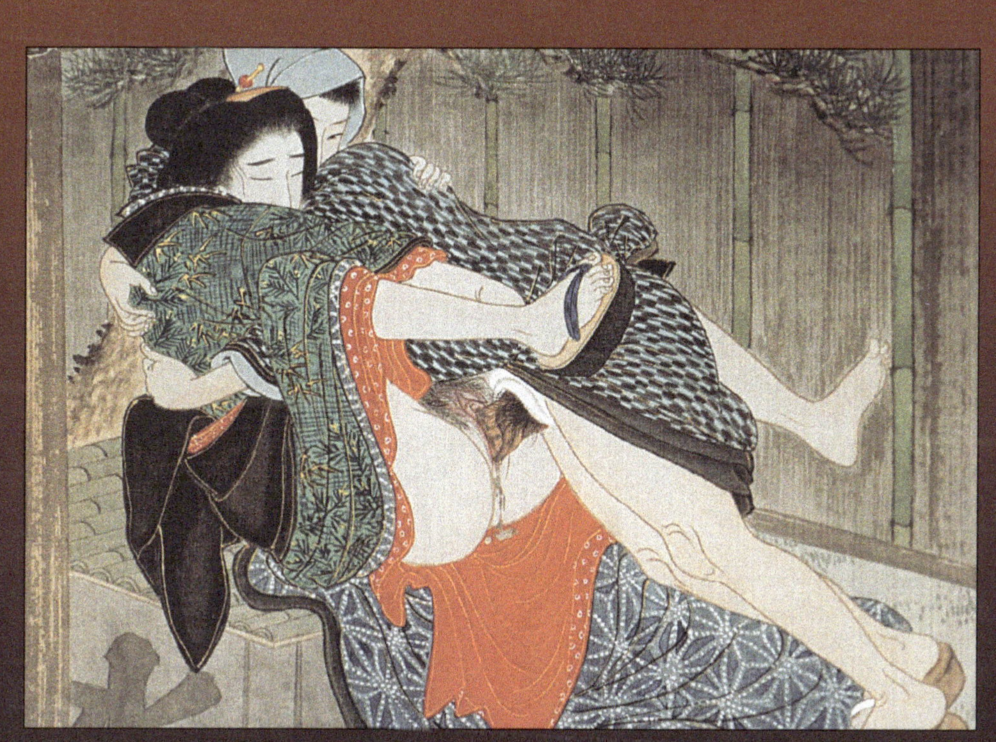

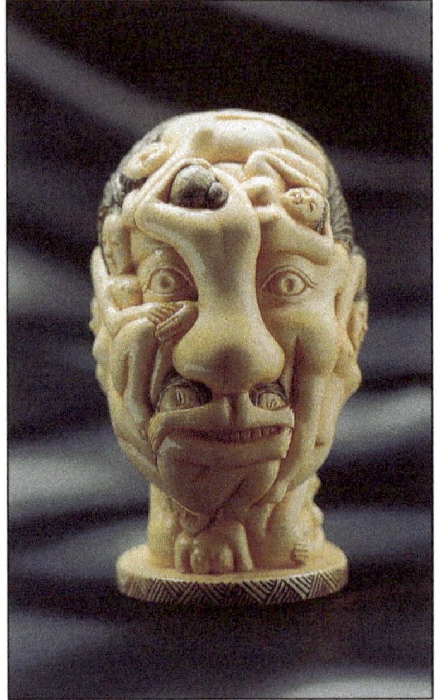

90

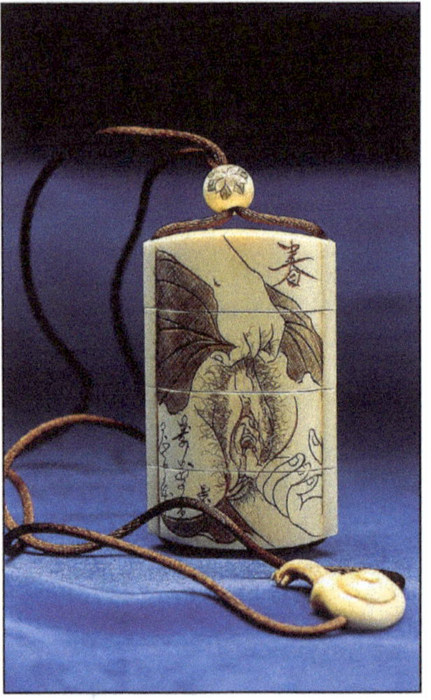

By contrast, in Japan throughout the 19th century these prints were hidden and forbidden. As the land of the rising sun became more industrialized, it also became more open to western influences and the Ukiyo-e disappeared into people's desk drawers. In effect, from the moment when the Meiji emperors seized power in 1868, Japan started flirting with the idea of assimilating into Europe. For this reason, any over-obvious signs of fertility cults or their symbols, especially images of the phallus, were suppressed as they were considered unworthy of a modern nation. The American occupation after the Second World War dealt the final blow to Shintoism. Today, most of the classical shungas which are offered for sale in the West are bought by Japanese collectors who in this way are returning them to their home country.

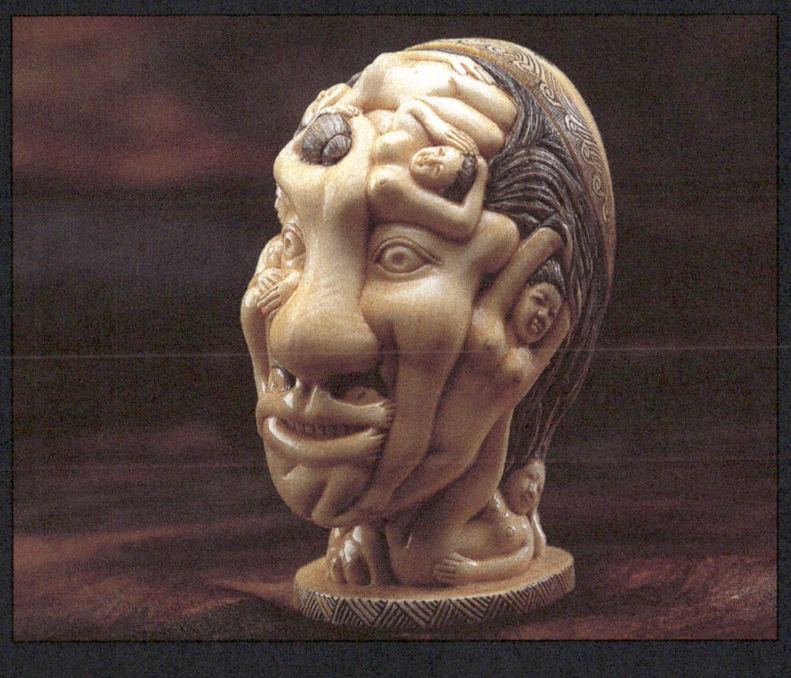

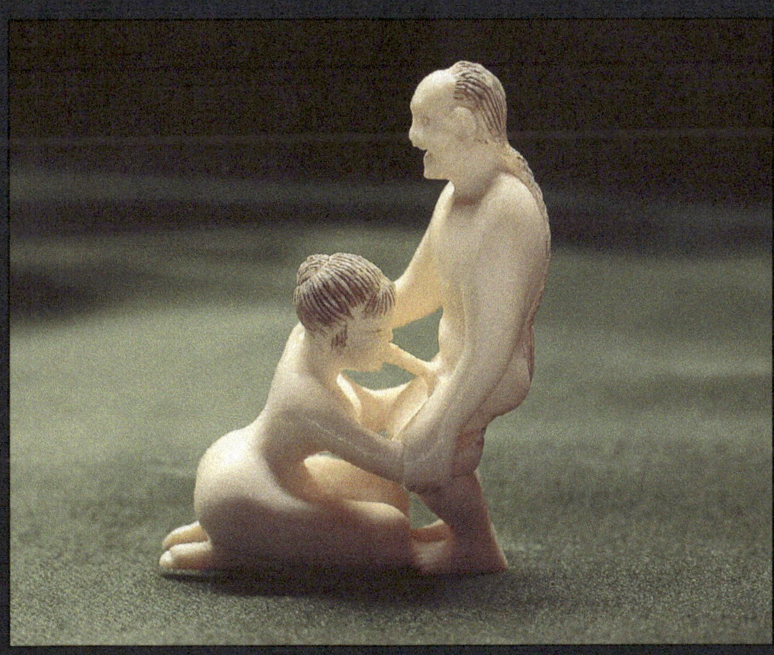

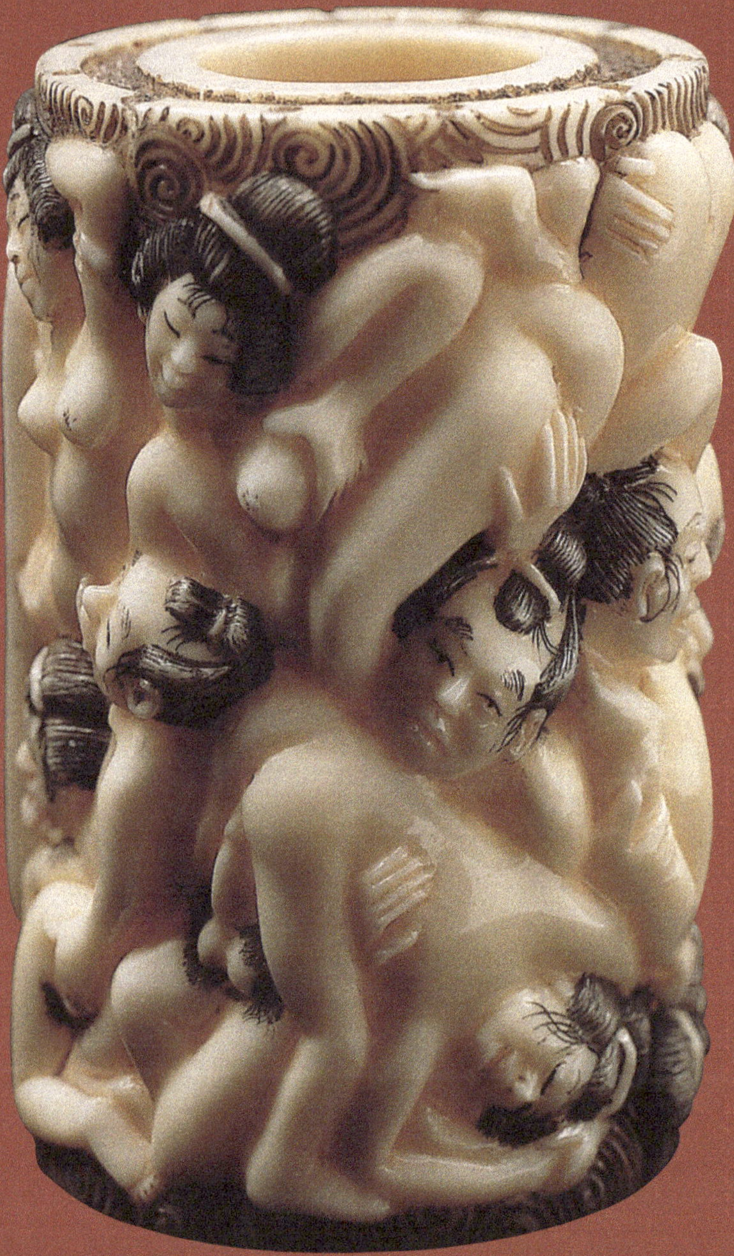

92

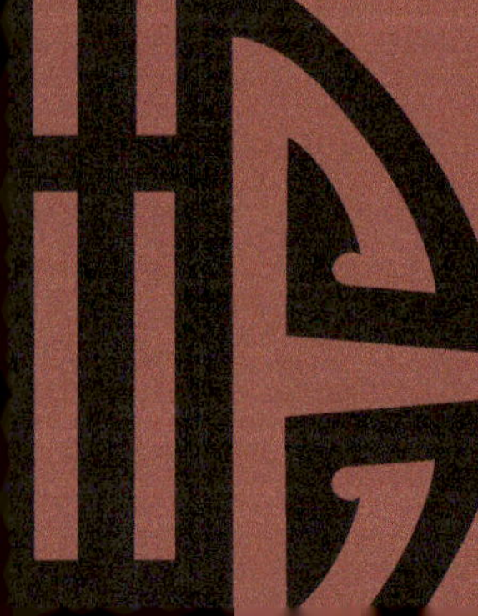

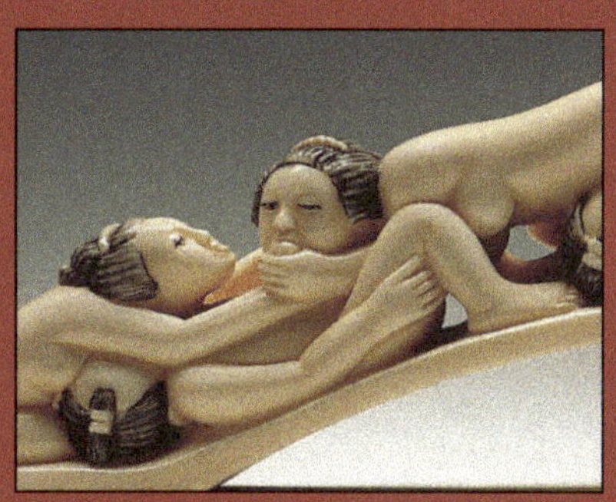

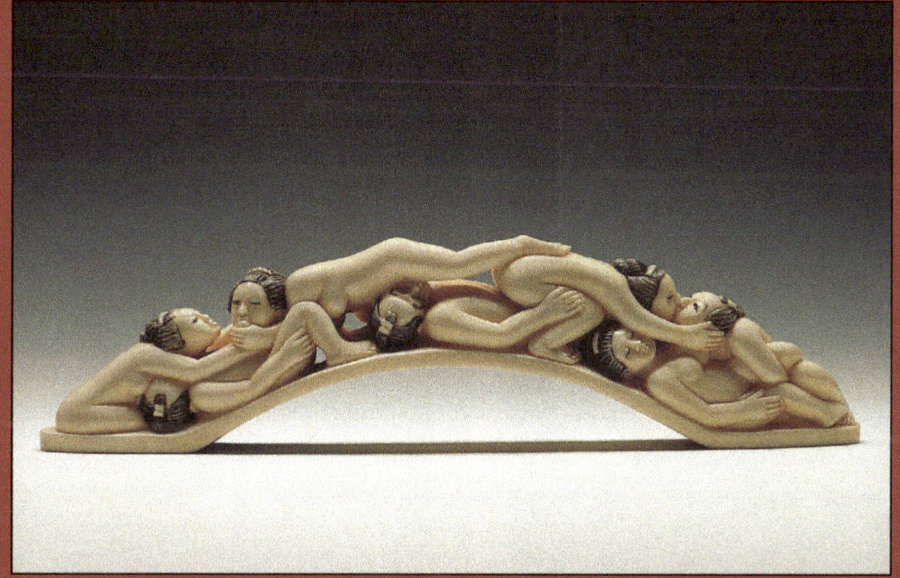

93

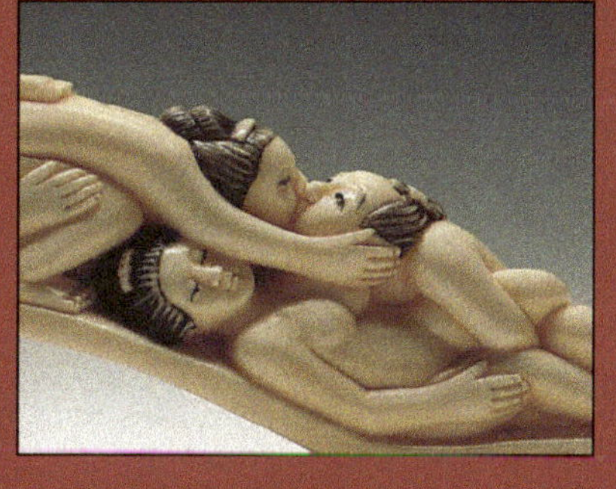

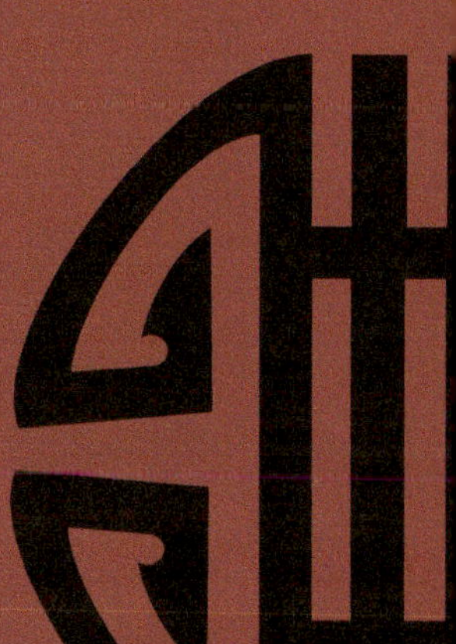

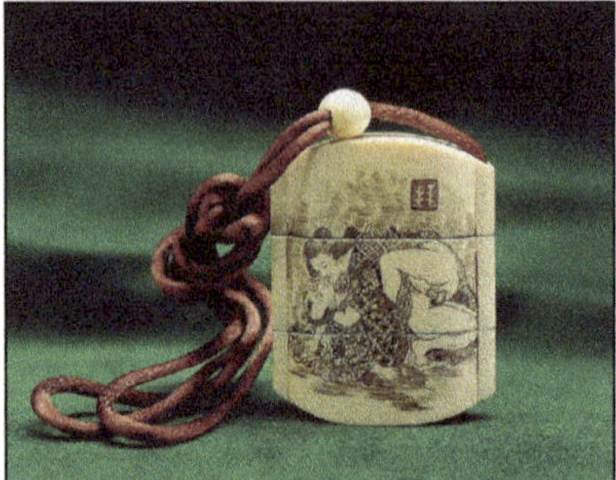

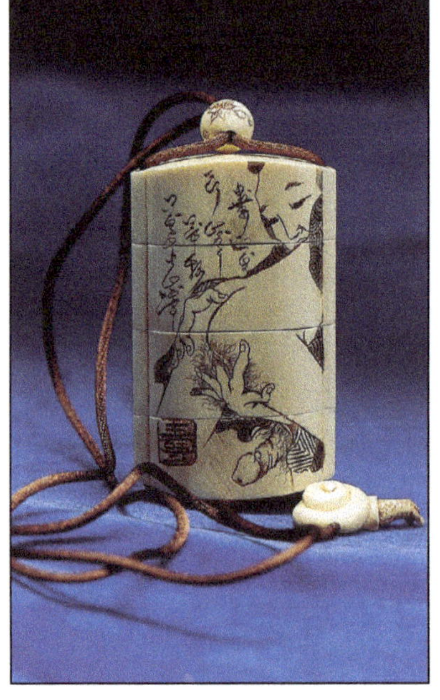

94

However, it was not until a massive exhibition of Japanese woodcarvings took place in 1973 in London, at the Victoria and Albert Museum, that the majority of art lovers were given the opportunity of relearning how to appreciate the true value of these erotic works.

Perhaps today we need to look at these works with new eyes, forgetting that over almost 150 years they served as the languorous representations of our desire for a simple sexuality that rises above all notion of 'sin'.

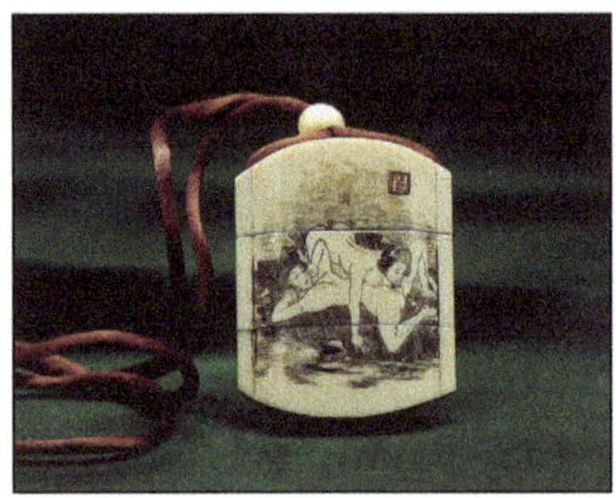

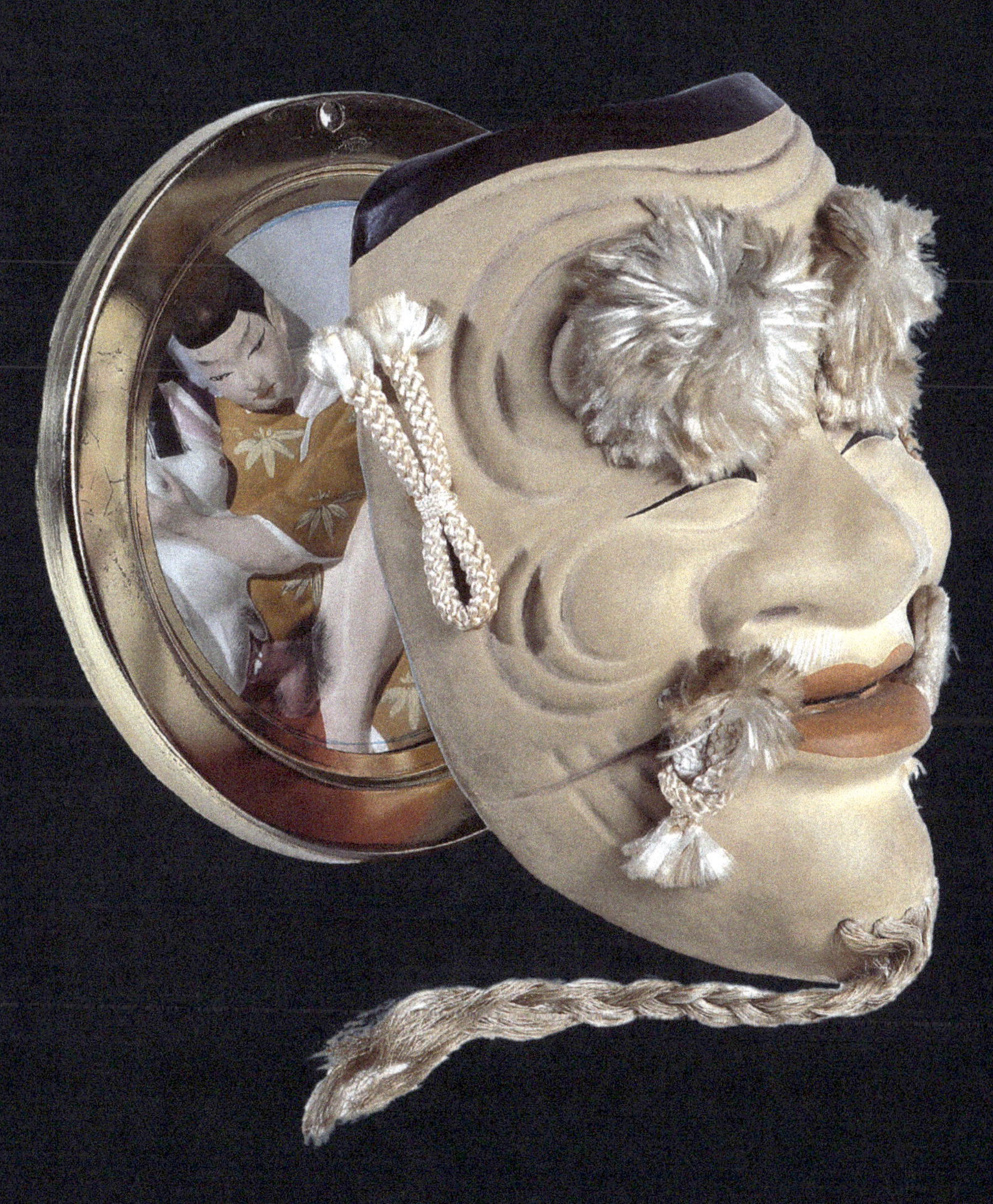

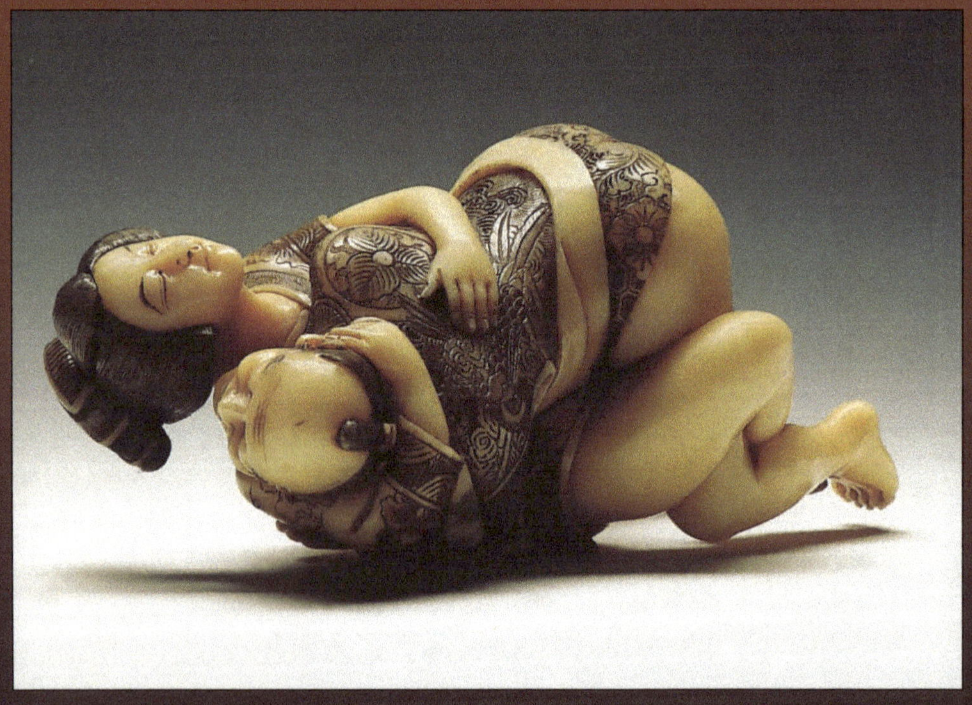

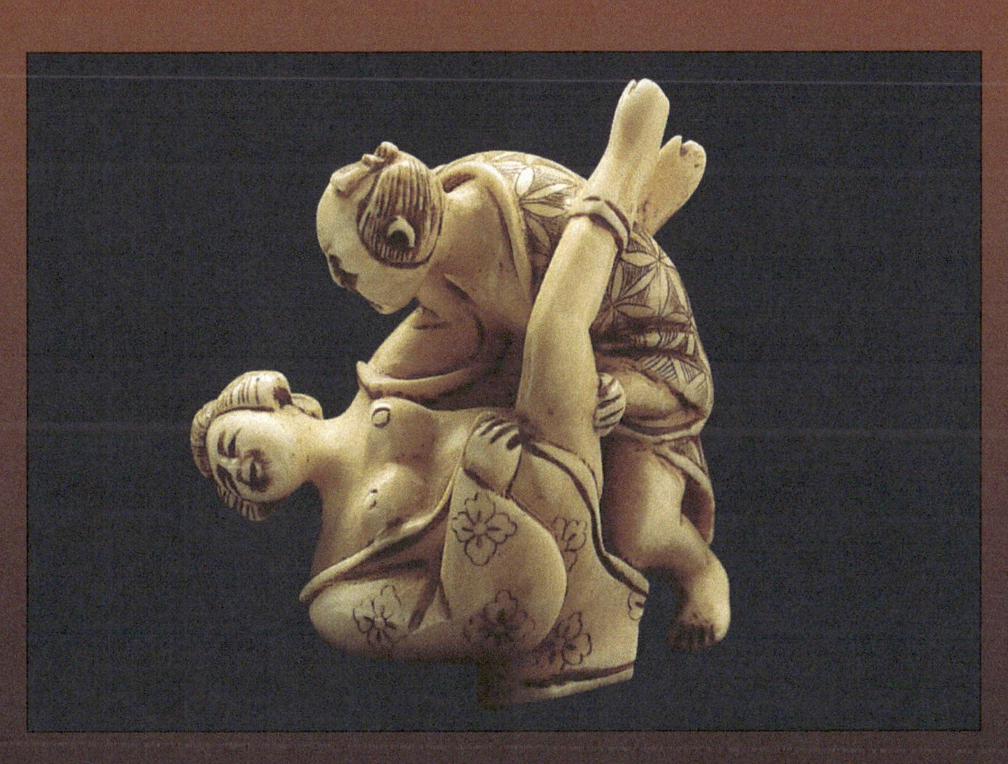

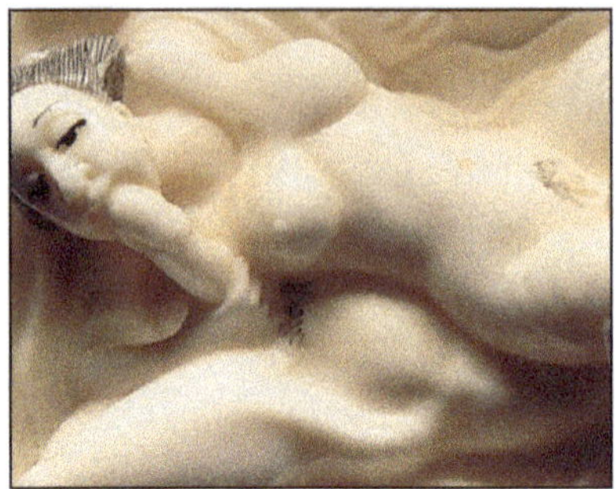

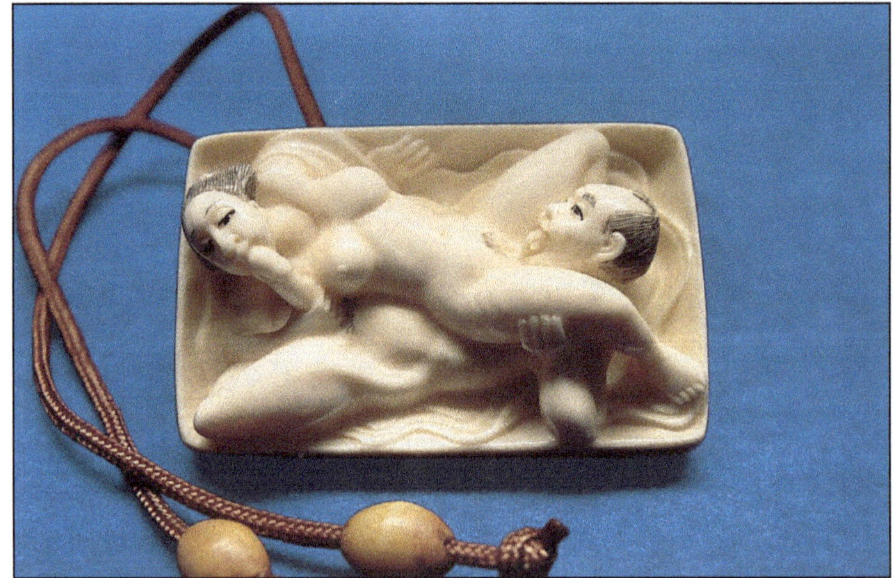

98

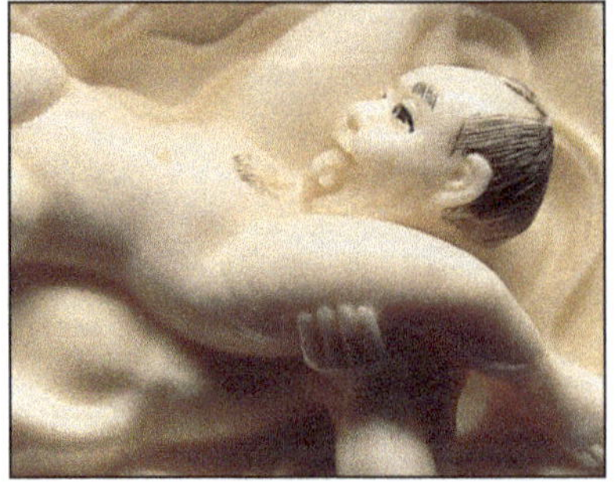

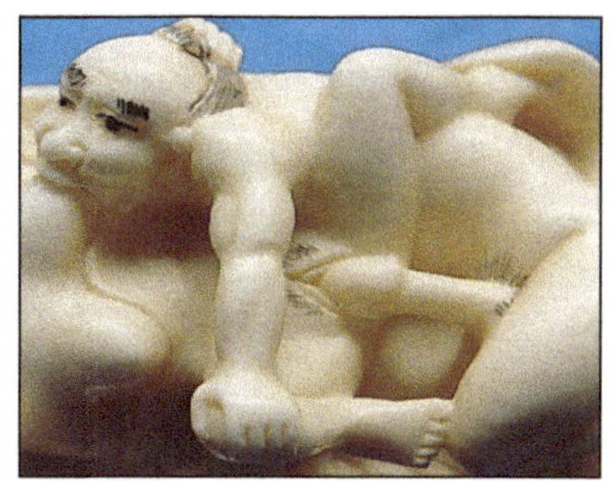

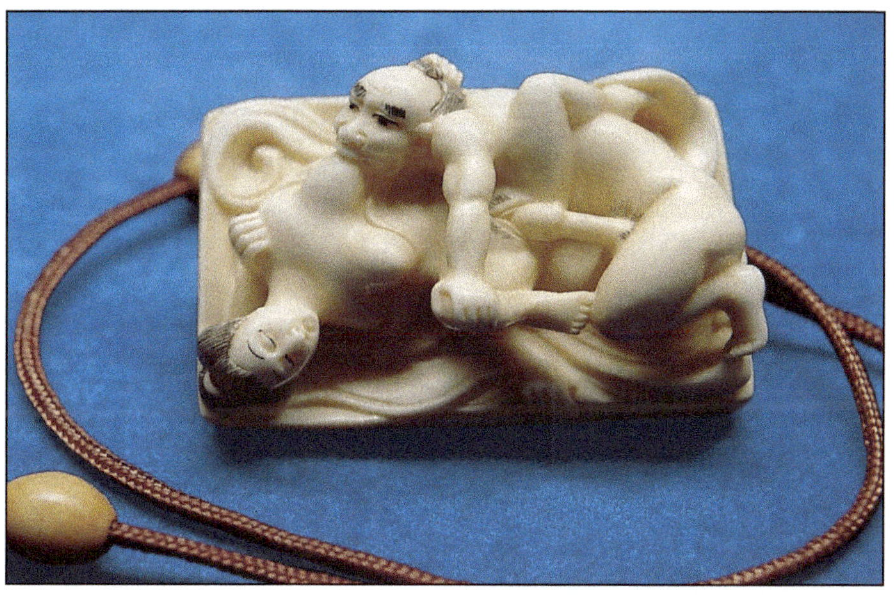

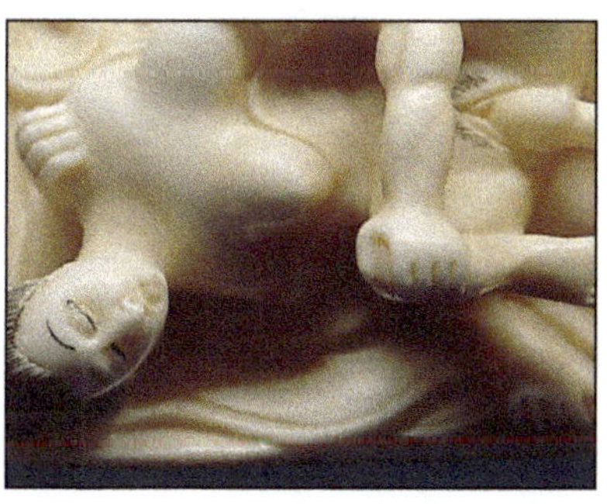

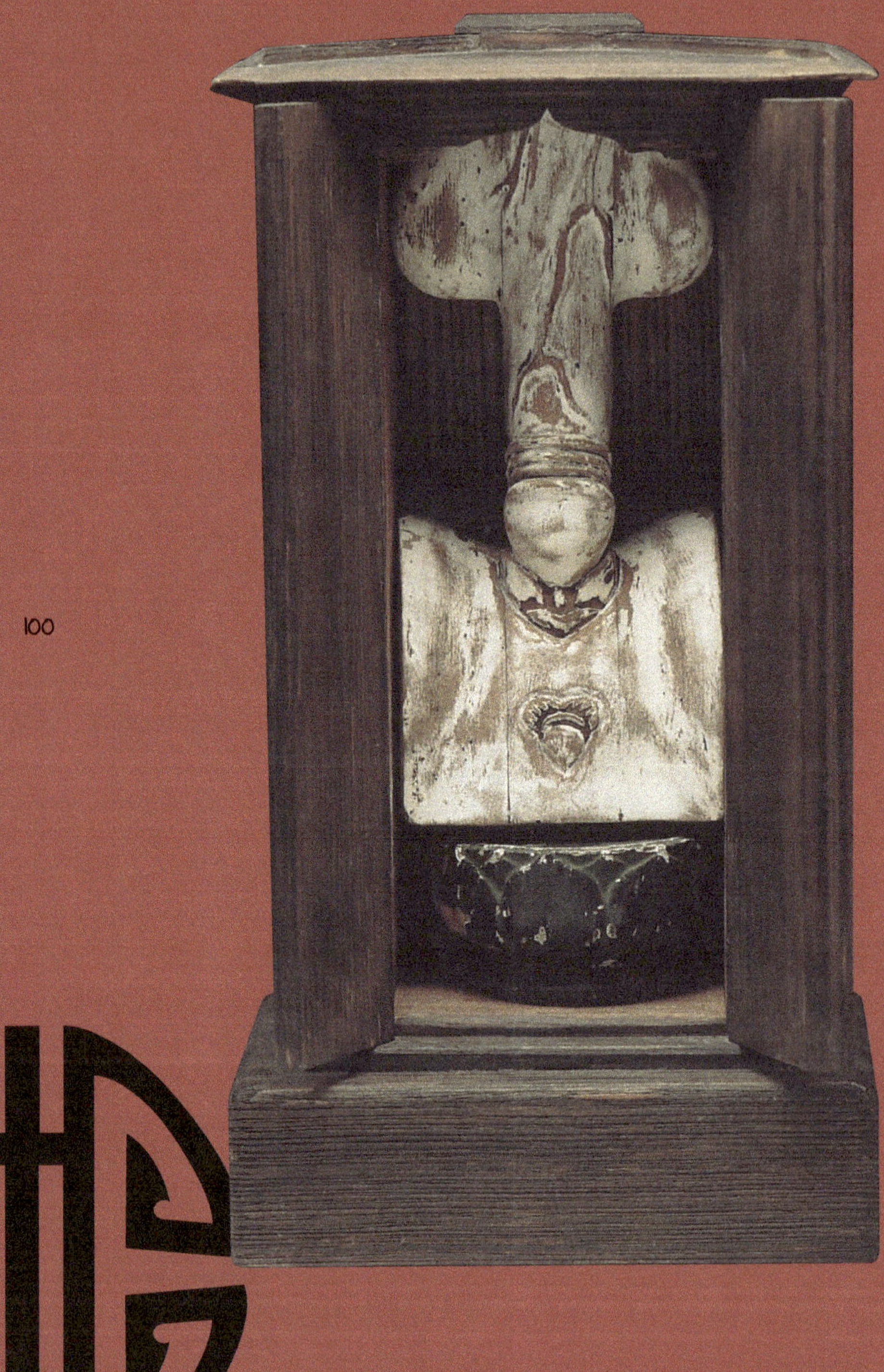

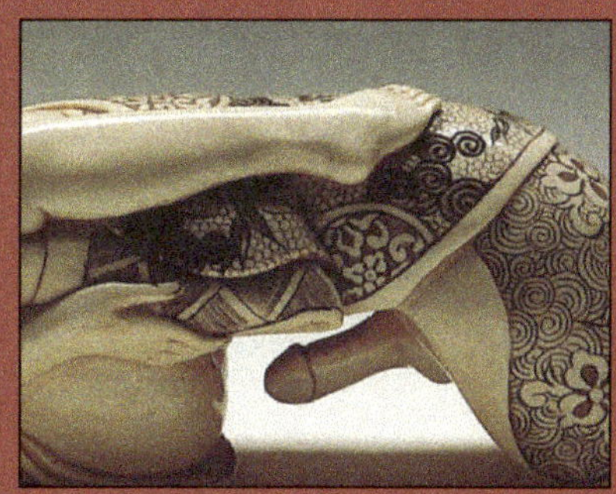

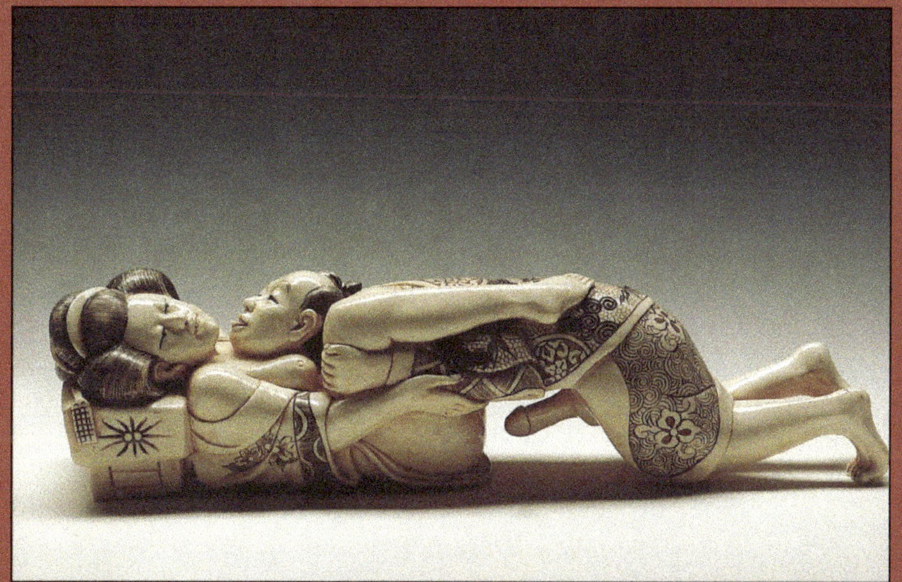

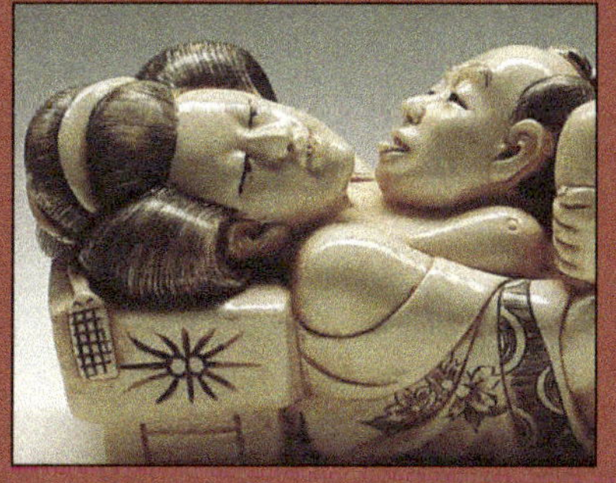

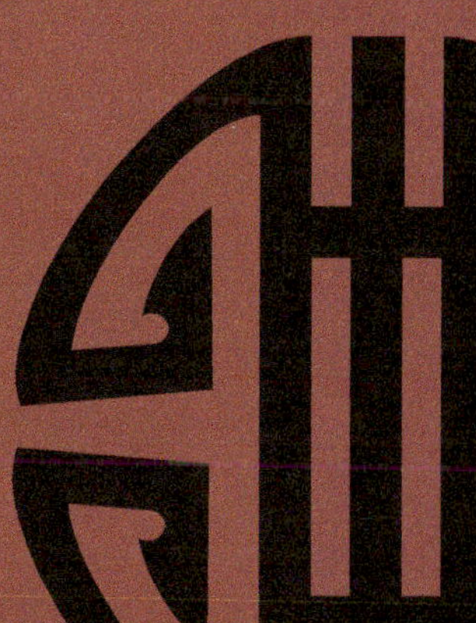

Chinese Eroticism

4–27: These images painted on silk derive from various marriage-books.
The 'marriage-books' of the 18th and 19th centuries were delicate and expensive volumes illustrating the different basic positions for love-making. Such a book was presented to daughters of the richest Chinese families on the day before their wedding, and represented a means of last-minute sexual education.

28: Two ornamental caskets, China, beginning of the 20th century. Top: *The Game of the Cloud and the Rain.* Bottom: Lesbian pair enjoying themselves with a dildo.

29: Monkey-nut in porcelain, China, end of the 19th century. Inside it is a couple making love, carved in a hard wood. The monkey-nut symbolizes fertility.

30-31: Top and bottom: Amorous couples, in Chinese porcelain, around 1900.

30-31: Center: Fruits, in Chinese porcelain, concealing a couple making love, around 1920.

32: Amorous couple in a boat propelled by two ducks. Engraved on ivory, around 1920.
Below: Snuffbox in painted porcelain, around 1920.

33: *The Charitable Deed*, sculpted in 18th-century style, varnished terracotta.

34-35: Couple making love, Chinese porcelain, around 1900.

36: Three ivory phalluses of different lengths usable as dildoes; 19th century.

37: Box featuring erotic images painted on glass.

38-39: Fruits, in Chinese porcelain, with a couple making love inside, around 1920.

Japanese Eroticism

42-89, 102:	Japanese *shunga* ("Images of Springtime"), 18th and 19th centuries. The *shunga* are specifically intended to emphasize the pleasures of the flesh.
90, 94:	*Inro* (Japanese belt-buckles) featuring engraved erotic scenes, modern.
90-91:	Top: Ivory bust in the style of Archimboldo, aggregating a number of models. Removing the top reveals an amorous couple beneath. Bottom: Fellatio, engraved on ivory, 20th century.
92:	Mass orgy, engraved on an ivory cylinder, modern.
93:	Seven figurines together representing an orgy, engraved on ivory, modern.
95:	Japanese theatrical mask. The face of the mask conceals an erotic motif on the back; 20th century.
96-97:	Japanese ivory figurines, around 1920.
98-99:	Netsuke, couples playing the game of love, 20th century.
100:	Fertility casket, Japan, 18th century, consecrated to Ko-jin, god of good fortune. The lotus is the symbol of the Creator Deity, thus also the symbol of purity and rebirth.
101:	Amorous couple, engraved on ivory, around 1920.
103:	Vase decorated with *shunga* motifs, modern copy.

Layout:
Baseline Co. Ltd
Ho-Chi-Minh-City, Vietnam

© 2020 Parkstone Press International, New York, USA
© 2020 Confidential Concepts, worldwide, USA
© **Image-Bar** www.image-bar.com

ISBN: 978-1-64699-167-9

Printed